Difference and IDENTITY

Difference and IDENTITY

A Special Issue of *Literature and Medicine*

Edited by
Jonathan M. Metzl and Suzanne Poirier

The Johns Hopkins University Press

Baltimore

© 2005 The Johns Hopkins University Press
All rights reserved. Published 2005
Printed in the United States of America
9 8 7 6 5 4 3 2 1

The Johns Hopkins University Press
2715 North Charles Street
Baltimore, Maryland 21218-4363
www.press.jhu.edu

Library of Congress Cataloging-in-Publication Data
Difference and identity : a special issue of Literature and medicine / edited by
Jonathan M. Metzl and Suzanne Poirier.
p. ; cm.
Includes bibliographical references.
ISBN 0-8018-8205-2 (pbk. : alk. paper)
1. Social medicine. 2. People with disabilities—Psychology. 3. Disabilities—Social
aspects. 4. AIDS (Disease)—Risk factors. 5. Human body—Social aspects. 6. Medicine
in literature. 7. Sex (Psychology)
[DNLM: 1. Medicine in Literature—Essays. 2. Cultural Characteristics—Essays.
3. Disabled Persons—psychology—Essays. 4. Health Knowledge, Attitudes,
Practice—Essays. 5. Sexual Behavior—psychology—Essays. 6. Stereotyping—Essays.
WZ 330 D569 2005] I. Metzl, Jonathan, 1964– II. Poirier, Suzanne. III. Literature
and medicine.
RA418.D498 2005
362.1'0422—dc22   2005009013

A catalog record for this book is available from the British Library.

For more information about *Literature and Medicine,* please see
www.press.jhu.edu/journals/literature_and_medicine.

CONTENTS

Preface: Difference and Identity in Medicine

Jonathan M. Metzl and Suzanne Poirier

Calls from within the field of medicine have asked nurses, doctors, and other health-care workers to become more aware of matters of difference. "[B]ias in health care must be corrected not by medical ombudsmen, or by legislation . . . but by a focus on the individual—individual patients and individual doctors," Abraham Verghese writes in the article "Showing Doctors Their Biases."[1] Mary Lebreck Kelley and Virginia Macken Fitzsimons's work teaches nurses to understand cultural diversity in clinical practice.[2] Medical humanities programs promote awareness of the social aspects of medicine, and the Association of American Medical Colleges has recently instituted cultural competencies for clinical interaction for the training of medical students.

These are timely and much-needed developments. Yet current efforts to impart understandings of the cultural and cross-cultural aspects of medicine suffer from an important limitation: within a medical system whose currency is diagnosis, difference is often defined through disease. Medical students learn, for instance, that African Americans are more likely to suffer from sickle-cell anemia, that women have a propensity for osteoporosis, and that schizophrenia preferentially afflicts the poor.

This special issue of *Literature and Medicine* focuses on difference and identity in the context of disease and disability. We explore the complex ways in which notions of disease, disability, and difference are intimately related and in which bodies marked by particular gender, racial, disability, sexuality, and ethnic identities experience disease in specific ways. Behind our investigation lies an assumption that understanding cultures and cultural ideologies is central to understanding bodies and diseases. For instance, osteoporosis is complicated by a number of factors that cannot be explained by individual pathology alone. Access to nutritional resources, cultural dietary practices, and types of labor all influence the manifestation, duration, and even the visibility of the disease. As another example, the different definitions of epilepsy between Hmong and American cultures, as described in Anne Fadiman's *The Spirit Catches You and You Fall Down*, arise from divergent assumptions about religion, wellness, disease, spirit, and soul. In her account, the Western medical establishment's inability to recognize these differences frustrates the well-intentioned efforts of doctors and nurses to treat a Hmong child.[3]

We acknowledge and build upon recent efforts of scholars in the social sciences to examine the centrality of identity to constructions of illness and health.[4] Yet the essays in this issue take decidedly humanities-based approaches to the subject in order to emphasize an awareness of and sensitivity to difference through forms of symbolic representation such as metaphor and narrative. The authors of these essays promote exploration of cultural assumptions about values, normality, and deviance while enabling appreciation for the particular and the idiosyncratic. Taken together, this issue highlights how the humanities are particularly adept at enhancing qualities that all good clinicians must possess in abundance: imagination and the inner resources to confront the unexpected. Along the way, we hope readers will learn to negotiate what academic psychiatrists Alexander Ortega and Robert Rosenheck call the effect of matters of difference "on symptom presentation" and to realize how beliefs about difference shape their own diagnostic perceptions.[5]

One way that the essays in this volume promote new understandings of difference and identity is through the exploration of visual knowledge. Medicine would not be what it is today without a long history of its concepts and competencies being presented, regularized, and disseminated visually. From Chinese acupuncture charts, to Vesalius's anatomical illustrations, to contemporary MRI scans, medical personnel have used images to train their eyes and sharpen their diagnostic capabilities, all the while acquiring sophisticated skill at interpreting and deploying visual cues. Yet the work of making sense of an image requires more than a mere recording of facts. For example, the knowledge required for comprehending images such as a Chinese yin-yang symbol or an American ultrasound scan depends upon the intricate interplay of history, experience, cultures of representation, and many other factors that help shape modalities of seeing. Scholars such as Sue Sun Yom, Stephen Rachman, Robert Goler, and Sander Gilman tap into this process, in which seeing always includes interpreting, in order to interrogate how visual information can mark differences of race, gender, body type, religion, or ethnicity. These authors call on

fields such as art history, film studies, and American studies in order
to unpack ideologies involved in the articulation and explanation of
images and representational systems. Along the way, their essays teach
readers to become more knowledgeable viewers and to reflect upon
the implications of their own positions as spectators.

Another focus of the essays in this volume is the representation
of medicine through textual narratives. Writing is a critical, though
sometimes overlooked, aspect of medicine, be it in a patient's chart, a
research report on a novel case, a popular article discussing a health
issue, an individual's account of his/her experiences with the health
system, or a personal description of an illness. Verghese's *My Own
Country: A Doctor's Story of a Town and Its People in the Age of AIDS*
about life in modern American medicine, Fanny Burney's account of
her mastectomy in early nineteenth-century Paris, a Yoruba mythologi-
cal tale explaining the origins of disease, Meri Nana-Ama Danquah's
Willow Weep for Me: A Black Woman's Journey Through Depression, and
Irvin Yalom's *Love's Executioner and Other Tales of Psychotherapy* are but
a few examples of the kinds of medical narratives produced within a
variety of cultural settings.[6] Oliver Sacks, as is well known, has used
narrative and the perspective of the individual as critical components of
his clinical diagnoses. Documents as standardized as hospital charts are
sites where rhetorical decisions about what to include or exclude—be
it the patient's temperature or his/her way of responding to persons
in authority—can shape the nature of the clinical interaction and responses to therapeutic interventions. Addressing this complexity, essays
by Tobin Siebers, Susan Squier, Gregory Tomso, David Kirby, and Lisa
Diedrich work to uncover how various forms of storytelling are neither
historically neutral nor purely individual but rather call upon conventions, genres, and other forms of culturally based modes of expression.
Their essays promote awareness of the multiplicity of perspectives and
points of view involved in a range of intimate, impersonal, or banal
interactions—from boarding an airplane, to unprotected sex, to visiting
a physician, to solitary meditation.

History is unfortunately replete with instances in which persons
have been pathologized and stigmatized based on externally imposed
misperceptions of difference or identity. "Diseases" from hysteria to
hypertension to homosexuality, among many others, have been critiqued
by historians and clinicians alike for institutionalizing cultural biases
as pathologies. As one example of such a critique, Sander Gilman's
essay describes how medical understandings of "[w]hat is considered
fat and what obese" have shifted over the course of time in response

to ever-changing and highly contextual notions of an "ideal" body weight. Yet, the essays in this volume work to the opposite effect—to lay claim to the agency of difference and, in the process, expose the ideologies and value judgments of the mainstream. They dissect the anatomy of a hegemonic "common sense" mentality, to cite David Kirby's discussion of Antonio Gramsci, in which categories of inside and outside, normal and deviant, are formed through subjective consent as much as through objective truth.

Although readers will no doubt find that these essays resonate with each other in even more ways than just described, we have grouped them together to suggest broad categories of difference that our authors incorporate, co-opt, and write against: disability, dis-sexuality, and disembodiment. Each section is framed by a short response from a leading scholar whose reflections are meant to illuminate connections and disjunctures among the texts.

Section one explores identities that are constructed, claimed, as-signed, or imposed through the rhetoric of disability. In "Disability as Masquerade," Tobin Siebers reads disability studies through the lens of queer theory in order to interrogate the epistemology of a poten-tially different closet. "To pass or not to pass," he asks, "but do . . . narratives about disability illustrate the conventional understanding of keeping secrets about identity?" Siebers uses Joan Riviere's 1929 essay, "Womanliness as a Masquerade," contemporary notions of stigma, the Americans with Disabilities Act, the writings of Joe Grigely and of Irving Zola, and his own experiences of navigating crowded airplane aisles "on wobbly legs" in order to trouble conventional understanding of disabled identity. Siebers's notion of "invisible disabilities" resonates through Susan Squier's "Meditation, Disability, and Identity," which investigates the changes that meditation evokes in disability identity. Squier draws on memoirs by people with disabilities who meditate, accounts of meditation-based therapies for people who are ill and/or disabled, and her own experiences of both disability and meditation in order to explore ways in which meditation catalyzes a shift in the understanding of disability, which grows out of a changed conception of the self. Like Squier, Sander Gilman attends to the tensions between cognitive and corporeal forms of disability in "Fat as Disability: The Case of the Jews." For Gilman, shifting cultural and historical notions of obesity interweave with beliefs about matters such as race, religion, volition, addiction, disease, and masculinity. He asks, "Is obesity the end product of impairment or is it impairment itself? If it is impairment, what organ is 'impaired'?" In his response, Thomas Laqueur brings into focus the social and political implications of disability claims by pointing out the almost unavoidable conflicts between disabled identities and the "categories under which an individual can make claims on the state for medical care, for legal protection, for pensions, for workman's compensation."

Section two treats the interactions of difference, identity, and sexuality. In "Bug Chasing, Barebacking, and the Risks of Care," Gregory Tomso analyzes a form of gay, HIV-positive sex that waves a certain flag at the world. Neither condoning nor condemning practices of unprotected sex, Tomso examines popular representations of bug chasing and barebacking as a way of gaining deeper access to popular and professional debates over the meanings of gay sexuality and epidemic disease. Sue Sun Yom's "Where the Girls Are: The Management of Venereal Disease by United States Military Forces in Vietnam" is also concerned with the rhetoric of promiscuity, only Sun focuses on a promiscuity that was tacitly encouraged even as it was officially maligned. For Sun, military-sponsored sexual-education films serve as an important introduction into the culture of the American military campaign in Vietnam. She shows how, beneath a rhetoric of public health and education, these films sexualize and reinforce the unequal social and economic power relations between American men and Vietnamese women. The duality of a sexuality that gives its subjects voice and mortally wounds them is also Lisa Diedrich's concern in "'Without us all told': Paul Monette's Vigilant Witnessing to the AIDS Crisis." Diedrich engages with the work of Timothy Murphy, Kelly Oliver, and other scholars of witnessing in order to read Monette's individual and highly personal testimonial of a mass epidemic. "We, the readers of Monette's work," Diedrich writes, "are . . . implicated in this process of witnessing; we too must cultivate our response-ability through our reading (at the very least) to those whom our society, in the age of AIDS, has made 'other.'" In her lyrical response, Sidonie Smith considers how the discourse of sexuality plays into the contemporary regime of human rights "and the identities and differences that regime sets in motion."

Finally, section three investigates differences and identities of embodiment. The section's first two essays find common ground in the aesthetics and multiple meanings surrounding nineteenth-century representations of deformity. Stephen Rachman's "Memento Morbi: Lam Qua's Paintings, Peter Parker's Patients" examines a remarkable series of 114 paintings made between 1836 and 1852 by the Cantonese artist Lam Qua depicting the Chinese patients of the medical missionary, Rev.

Dr. Peter Parker. The essay addresses the ways in which Lam Qua's representations of patients with "mature tumors" serve as complex documents of cultural confluence and exchange between "East and West, Orient and Occident, portraiture and clinical documentation, Christian and heathen, rich and poor." A continent and a world away, Robert Goler's "Loss and the Persistence of Memory: 'The Case of George Dedlow' and Disabled Civil War Veterans" examines the cultural meanings attributed to the American Civil War's disabled veterans by analyzing representations of soldiers whose limbs were amputated as a result of battlefield injuries. Goler uses S. Weir Mitchell's 1866 short story, "The Case of George Dedlow," and the postwar discourse of amputation to discern shifting narratives of national trauma, personal trauma, and "the symbolic role assigned veteran amputees in the search for communal suture." David Kirby's "Extrapolating Race in *GATTACA*: Genetic Passing, Identity, and the Science of Race" moves from past to future, and from body to disembodiment, through an analysis of the human-gene technologies imagined in science fiction cinema. For Kirby, the 1997 science fiction film *GATTACA* serves as a jumping-off point for a discussion of the racialized underpinnings of a world in which "a person's only sense of identity comes from his or her genes." In his response essay, Joel Howell ties the rhetoric of "distorted and absent body parts" to that of "idealized and perfect body parts" while considering "the tension between lofty ideals and the inherent messiness of life, of medicine, and of health care."

The editors of this special issue extend thanks to the authors, reviewers, and editorial staff for their limitless energy, flexibility, and dedication. The project arose out of a University of Michigan faculty initiative in Culture, Health, and Medicine, which was funded by the United States Department of Education's Fund for the Improvement of Postsecondary Education (FIPSE) program.[7] Additional support came from the Michigan Life Sciences, Values, and Society Program.

Of course, our topic selection in no way exhausts the many complex ways that notions of difference and identity impact constructions of illness and health. Rather, in unique and creative ways, each essay in this issue provides a heuristic lens through which to consider the relationships between individual expressions of identity and communal experiences of difference. Each piece also speaks to the process whereby individual stories and strategies shape, and are in turn shaped by, the institutions they seek to transform. "The epistemology of the closet complicates the usual understanding of passing," Tobin Siebers writes in his essay, "because it disrupts the structural binary that represents passing as an action taking place between knowing and unknowing subjects." In understanding the narratives of others, in other words, we ultimately learn to rethink ourselves.

NOTES

1. Abraham Verghese, "Showing Doctors Their Biases," *New York Times*, March 1, 1999, A21.

2. Mary Lebreck Kelley and Virginia Macken Fitzsimons, *Understanding Cultural Diversity: Culture, Curriculum, and Community in Nursing* (Sudbury, MA: Jones and Bartlett, 2000).

3. Anne Fadiman, *The Spirit Catches You and You Fall Down: A Hmong Child, Her American Doctors, and the Collision of Two Cultures* (New York: Farrar, Straus and Giroux, 1998).

4. Cathy Cohen, *The Boundaries of Blackness: AIDS and the Breakdown of Black Politics* (Chicago: University of Chicago Press, 1999); Kimberlé Crenshaw, "Mapping the Margins: Intersectionality, Identity Politics, and Violence Against Women of Color," in *Critical Race Theory: The Key Writings that Formed the Movement*, ed. K. Crenshaw et al. (New York: New Press, 1995), 357–83; Edna Viruell-Fuentes and Leslie R. Wolfe, *"Telling My Story"—Women with HIV Speak Out About Their Lives* (Washington, DC: Center for Women Policy Studies, 1998).

5. Alexander Ortega and Robert Rosenheck, "Posttraumatic Stress Disorder among Hispanic Vietnam Veterans," *American Journal of Psychiatry* 157, no. 4 (2000): 615–9. "The study of mental disorders among Hispanics presents numerous methodological challenges, such as . . . the need to assess the differential effect of ethnocultural factors on symptom presentation and community functioning" (615).

6. Abraham Verghese, *My Own Country: A Doctor's Story of a Town and Its People in the Age of AIDS* (New York: Vintage Books, 1995); Fanny Burney to Esther Burney, Paris, 30 September 1811, in *The Journals and Letters of Fanny Burney* (Madame D'Arblay), ed. Joyce Hemlow et al. (Oxford: Clarendon Press, 1975), 596–616; Meri Nana-Ama Danquah, *Willow Weep for Me: A Black Woman's Journey Through Depression* (New York: One World, 1999); and Irvin D. Yalom, *Love's Executioner and Other Tales of Psychotherapy* (New York: Basic Books, 1989).

7. For more information about this initiative, visit http://www.umich.edu/

Difference and IDENTITY

Disability as Masquerade
Tobin Siebers

I.

My subject will be recognized as passing although I plan to give
it a few unexpected twists and turns. For I have been keeping secrets
and telling lies. In December 1999, I had an altercation at the San
Francisco airport with a gatekeeper for Northwest Airlines, who demanded that I use a wheelchair if I wanted to claim the early-boarding
option. He did not want to accept that I was disabled unless my status
was validated by a highly visible prop like a wheelchair. In the years
since I have begun to feel the effects of postpolio, my practice has been
to board airplanes immediately after the first-class passengers so that I
do not have to navigate crowded aisles on wobbly legs. I answered the
gatekeeper that I would be in a wheelchair soon enough, but that it was
my decision, not his, when I began to use one. He eventually let me
board and then chased after me on an afterthought to apologize. The
incident was trivial in many ways, but I have now adopted the habit
of exaggerating my limp whenever I board planes. My exaggeration is
not always sufficient to render my disability visible—gatekeepers still
question me on occasion—but I continue to use the strategy, despite the
fact that it fills me with a sense of anxiety and bad faith, emotions that
resonate with previous experiences in which doctors and nurses have
accused me of false complaints, oversensitivity, and malingering.

In January 2001, I slipped on a small patch of ice and broke my
knee. It was my right knee, the leg affected by polio when I was two
years old. For the next few months, I used wooden crutches, a prosthetic device, unlike forearm crutches, that usually signifies temporary
injury rather than long-term disability. Throughout my life I have spent
long periods on crutches, and my return to them summoned a series
of powerful emotions. For one thing, it was the first time I found myself
on crutches since I had come out as disabled.[1] The crutches projected
to the public world what I felt to be a profound symbol of my inner
life as well as my present status as a person with a disability. They also

1

gave me great hope for the future because I had begun to worry that I would not be able to get around as I grew older, and I soon realized to my relief that I could do very well on my crutches. I had been tutored in their use from such an early age that I felt as if a part of my body once lost to me had somehow been restored as soon as I slipped them under my arms. Nevertheless, I found myself giving an entirely new answer to the question posed to me by people on the street. "What's wrong with you?" they always ask. My new answer: "I slipped on the ice and broke my knee."

To pass or not to pass—that is often the question. But do these two narratives about disability illustrate the conventional understanding of keeping secrets about identity? Erving Goffman defines passing as a strategy for managing the stigma of "spoiled identities"—those discredited by law, opinion, or social convention.[2] When in the minority and powerless, Jews pass as Christians, blacks pass as whites, and gay, lesbian, and transgendered people pass as heterosexuals. Similarly, people with disabilities find ingenious ways to conceal their impairments and pass as able-bodied. In *Epistemology of the Closet*, however, Eve Kosofsky Sedgwick suggests that secrets concerning identity are a more complicated affair than Goffman's definition allows, arguing persuasively that the historical specificity of the closet has marked indelibly the meaning of "secrecy" in twentieth-century Western culture.[3] Closeting involves things not merely concealed but difficult to disclose—the inability to disclose is, in fact, one of the constitutive markers of oppression. The epistemology of the closet complicates the usual understanding of passing because it disrupts the structural binary that represents passing as an action taking place between knowing and unknowing subjects. The closet often holds secrets that either cannot be told or are being kept by those who do not want to know the truth about the closeted person. Some people keep secrets; other people are secrets. Some people hide in the closet, but others are locked in the closet. There is a long history, of course, of locking away people with disabilities in attics, basements, and backrooms—not to mention the many institutions created to keep secret the existence of disabled family members. Secrets about disability may appear mundane compared to those associated with the gay experience because the closet cannot be mapped according to the simple binary opposition between private and public existence. But if disability studies has anything to learn from queer theory, it is that secrecy rarely depends on simple binaries.

Sedgwick argues that an open secret compulsorily kept characterizes the epistemology of the closet, and she provides as an example the bewildering case of an eighth-grade schoolteacher named Acanfora who disclosed his homosexuality and was removed from the classroom. When he sued the local board of education, a federal court found that he could not be denied employment because of his homosexuality but supported the decision of the board to remove him because he had not disclosed his homosexuality on his job application (69–70). By a tortured logic, too much information suddenly became too little, and Acanfora was punished. It is increasingly apparent that a similar logic also plagues disability law, which is one reason why queer theory holds important lessons for disability studies. In a recent high-profile case, the United States Supreme Court found that two women pilots denied employment by United Airlines because they were nearsighted could not seek protection under the Americans with Disabilities Act due to the fact that they were not disabled. The social representation of difference as negative or inferior, not the existence of physical and mental differences, defines disability discrimination. Yet the two pilots were not allowed to seek protection under the law, even though United Airlines denied them employment by deeming their bodies inferior and the Court ruled that this representation was false. For the purposes of the law, the women were given two bodies, one by the Court and another by United Airlines, as if doing so were the only way to sustain the impossible double standard being applied to them.[4]

The incoherent legal cases of Acanfora and the women pilots expose the closet at work, what Sedgwick calls "vectors of a disclosure at once compulsory and forbidden" (70). The closet is an oppressive structure because it controls the flow of information beyond individual desire for disclosure or secrecy and because it is able to convert either disclosure or secrecy into the opposite. Putting oneself in the closet is not as easy as closing the door. Coming out of the closet is not as simple as opening it. Parents and relatives do not want to hear about queer identity. "Don't Ask, Don't Tell" is, of course, the motto of the military.[5] Wheelchair users understand what it is to be overlooked by a sea of passersby, and people with birthmarks or facial deformities are often strategically ignored as well. The smallest facial deformity invites the furtive glance, stolen when you are not looking, looking away when you look back. Invite the stare you otherwise fear, and you may find yourself invisible, beyond staring.[6] Passing is possible not only because people have sufficient genius to disguise their identity but also because society has a general tendency to repress the embodiment of difference. This is what queer theory teaches people with disabilities about the epistemology of the closet.

Nevertheless, the closet may not be entirely adequate to portray the experience of people with disabilities. Sedgwick makes the case that the image of the closet, as resonant as it may be for many modern oppressions, is "indicative for homophobia in a way it cannot be for other oppressions," including "physical handicap" (75). Oppressions based on race, gender, age, size, and disability, according to Sedgwick, focus on visible stigmas, while homophobia does not.[7] The concept of visible stigma provides no good reason, I will argue, to dissociate disability from the epistemology of the closet because it does not take into account invisible disabilities such as deafness, chronic fatigue, autism, and dyslexia. More important, it makes no sense to link oppression to physical and mental characteristics of the body, visible or not, because the cause of oppression usually exists in the social or built environment and not in the body. Every inaccessible building is a closet representing the oppression of people with disabilities by able-bodied society. I do think, however, that Sedgwick is correct to hesitate about the wholesale equivalence of passing with regard to disability and homosexuality—not because people with disabilities are not closeted but because disability passing presents forms of legibility and illegibility that alter the logic of the closet.

Although people with disabilities may try to pass in the classic sense of the term by concealing their disability from discovery, they also engage in a little discussed practice, structurally akin to passing but not identical to it, in which they disguise one kind of disability with another or display their disability by exaggerating it. This practice clouds the legibility of passing, and it is sufficiently different from traditional passing both to merit a closer look and to invite its own terminology. My strategy here is to reach out to queer theory and its prehistory for models to think about both passing and the politicization of identity in the disability community. Nevertheless, my argument is meant to be "second wave" insofar as it is concerned less with passing in the classic sense than with unconventional uses of disability identity. My method is to gather as many narratives about alternative disability passing as possible to make up for the dearth of theory, since narrative is, according to Barbara Christian, where theory takes place.[8] I refer to these altered forms of disability passing as the "masquerade."

II.

The concept of the masquerade, long a staple of feminist and queer theory, offers an opportunity to rethink passing from the point of view of disability studies because it claims disability as a version of itself rather than simply concealing it from view. Joan Riviere's 1929 essay, "Womanliness as a Masquerade," presents the case study of a gifted academic who flirts compulsively with the men in her audience after each successful intellectual performance, wearing the mask of womanliness to defend herself against both her own feelings of gender anxiety and reprisals by men.[9] "I shall attempt to show," Riviere explains, "that women who wish for masculinity may put on a mask of womanliness to avert anxiety and retribution feared from men" (91). While this mask serves as a form of passing, it differs from the classic forms defined by queer theory and critical race studies. Gay, lesbian, bisexual, and transgendered people who closet themselves or people of color who pretend to be white usually wish to avoid social stigmatization and to gain the safety and advantages offered by dominant social roles. Only rarely do dominant groups try to pass as lesser ones. Adrian Piper, for example, notes that being black is a social condition that "no white person would voluntarily assume."[10] Passing preserves social hierarchies because it assumes that individuals want to rise above their present social station and that the station to which they aspire belongs to a dominant social group. It stamps the dominant social position as simultaneously normative and desirable.

Riviere's "woman," however, puts on a socially stigmatized identity as her disguise. She mimics neither the normative nor the dominant social position. She displays her stigma to protect herself from her own anxiety and reprisals by men, but she does not pass. In fact, Riviere leaves behind very quickly specific reference to the closet. She comes to the famous conclusion that there is no difference between "genuine womanliness" and the "masquerade." "Whether radical or superficial," Riviere writes, "they are the same thing" (94). In other words, straight and gay women alike (and some men) put on the mask of womanliness, despite the fact that it represents a spoiled identity or "undesired differentness," to apply Goffman's understanding of social stigma (5). Riviere is describing both the ideological pressures on women to subject themselves to men by performing weakness, passivity, and erotic receptivity as well as the unequal gender conditions and accompanying feelings of oppression motivating the performance.[11] The masquerade represents an alternative method of managing social stigma through disguise, one relying not on the imitation of a dominant social role but on the assumption of an identity marked as stigmatized, marginal, or inferior.

Joseph Grigely, a conceptual and visual artist, offers a parallel to the gender masquerade described by Riviere in his own desire at times to masquerade his deafness. He reacts to a recent experience at the Metropolitan Museum of Art where a guard struck him on the shoulder and berated him for not responding the first time to a command that he stop sitting on the floor: "I look into a mirror at myself, search for my deafness, yet fail to find it. For some reason we have been conditioned to presume difference to be a visual phenomenon, the body as the locus of race and gender. Perhaps I need a hearing aid, not a flesh-colored one but a red one . . . a signifier that ceremoniously announces itself."[12] Grigely feels compelled to out himself as disabled so that able-bodied people will not be confused, which guarantees at the same time that he will be rendered invisible. Drawing upon Adrienne Rich's concept of compulsory heterosexuality, we can interpret his feelings as a response to "compulsory able-bodiedness," a logic that presents the able body, according to Robert McRuer, as an ideological norm casting disability as the exception necessary to confirm that norm.[13] Hence the desire that people with disabilities sometimes experience to overcome their invisibility and its attendant violence by exhibiting their impairments, and the paradoxical consequence that they become even more invisible and vulnerable as a result. In fact, according to the logic of compulsory able-bodiedness, the more visible the disability, the greater the chance that the disabled person will be repressed from public view and forgotten. The masquerade shows that disability exists at the same time that it, as masquerade, does not exist.

Although Riviere sometimes stresses the use of the masquerade as a response to injustice and oppression, she tries at the same time to resist this conclusion in favor of a narrower psychoanalytic explanation. She gives the classic psychoanalytic reading of œdipal rivalry in which unresolved personal conflicts torment the individual with anxiety while providing a vivid picture of what it must have been like to be a woman competing with men in early twentieth-century intellectual circles. She is acutely aware of the closed nature of these circles, of the daily parade of potentially hostile doctors and lawyers faced by any woman who dared enter there, because she had direct experience of it in her own life. Moreover, her patient tells her that she bitterly resents "any assumption" that she is "not equal" to the men around her and rejects "the idea of being subject to their judgment or criticism" (93). Riviere, however, does not allow that feelings of inequality and rejection of them should figure as part of her patient's social reality.[14] Womanliness is merely a symptom of internal psychic conflicts originating in early family life.

More importantly, when Riviere makes the famous leap generalizing the masquerade as a condition of femininity, she must also generalize the situation of the woman in the case study. The woman is one among many women with this problem, potentially one among all women, for she displays "well-known manifestations of the castration complex" (97). The reference to castration is crucial because it introduces a slippage between the categories of woman and disabled person. The castrated body, though imaginary, is read as a disabled body, with the result that all women are figured by psychoanalysis as disabled.[15] Moreover, Riviere's description of her patient's underlying motives for the masquerade as "sadism," "rivalry," and the desire for "supremacy" attributes her behavior to psychological disability rather than political action or social protest (98–9).

"Rivalry" and the desire for "supremacy" are infelicitous formulations for the need to protest against inequality and subjugation. They remind one of phrases often used today to characterize marginalized groups as "schools of resentment" or as bound by "wounded attachments."[16] The problem is especially aggravating in the case of people with disabilities because their calls for justice have so often been dismissed as special pleading by selfish or resentful individuals who claim to be the exception to every rule and care nothing for what is best for the majority. Better to use a political vocabulary, I insist, that attacks assumptions of inequality and rejects the idea that one should be categorically subjected to others because of individual psychology or ability.[17]

III.

Successful political explanations avoid single and simple axioms in favor of respect for the complexity of human behavior. The world of politics will never be other than a messy place, no matter how much we think we know and how much experience we garner. If the reasons for disability masquerading are political, they cannot be reduced to simple laws but must be tracked through examples, descriptions, and narratives that establish greater awareness about the everyday existence of people with disabilities as well as attack the history of their misrepresentation. The task is not easy because there are few stories available told from the point of view of the disability community, and the desire to repress disability is powerful in our society. But if Tom Shakespeare is right, it is crucial to explore the range of possibilities defining disability identity. He argues that a qualitative difference exists between disability identities that claim disability and those that do not. Attempts to pass create temporary or compromised identities costly to individual happiness and safety while positive disability identities, often linked to "coming-out," reject oppression and seek to develop new narratives of the self and new political forms.[18]

Greater awareness about disability identity requires both the ability to abstract general rules on the basis of one's experience and to recognize that one's experience differs from that of others. The challenge is to find a rhetorical form that satisfies theoretical, practical, and political requirements. Narratives about disability identity are theoretical because they posit a different experience that clashes with how social existence is usually constructed and recorded. They are practical because they often contain solutions to problems experienced by disabled and nondisabled people alike. They are political because they offer a basis for identity politics, allowing people with different disabilities to tell a story about their common cause. The story of this common cause is also the story of a constitutive outside that reveals a great deal about what any given society contains. For example, when a disabled body moves into a social space, the lack of fit exposes the shape of the normative body for which the space was originally designed. Disabled identities make a difference, and in making this difference, they require a story that illuminates the society in which they are found.

Identities are a means of inserting persons into the social world. They are narrative responses to and creations of social reality, aiding cooperation between people, representing significant theories about the construction of the real, and containing useful information about how human beings should make their appearance in the world.[19] Disability identities would seem to be the exception to this rule: they are perceived as a bad fit, their relation to society is largely negative, and so, it would seem, is their theoretical value. In fact, the reverse may be true. While people with disabilities have little power in the social world, their identities possess great theoretical power because they reflect perspectives capable of illuminating the ideological blueprints used to construct social reality.[20] "Some identities," as Paula Moya puts it, "can be more politically progressive than others *not* because they are 'transgressive' or 'indeterminate' but because they provide us with a critical perspective from which we can disclose the complicated workings of ideology and oppression."[21]

The problem, of course, is to move from theoretical to political power, to find a way to use critical knowledge about society to effect political transformation. The masquerade, I have been suggesting, claims disability as a way to manage the stigma of social difference, but I will now tell stories about the politics of this strategy. The six narratives that follow are designed to provide a fuller, though still admittedly incomplete, description of the theoretical and political implications of disability masquerade. Each narrative takes the form of a fable, with the political moral appended at the beginning rather than the end of the story. Narratives one through four explore the benefits of the masquerade for people with disabilities. The fifth and sixth narratives show the disadvantages of this practice.

The masquerade may inflect private and public space, allowing expression of a public view of disability for political ends. Consider the example of the Capitol protest for the Americans with Disabilities Act in the spring of 1990. Three dozen wheelchair users, representing ADAPT (American Disabled for Accessible Public Transit, a public transportation advocacy group for people with disabilities), abandoned their chairs to crawl up the eighty-three marble steps of the Capitol building.[22] None of the protestors, I suspect, made a practice of crawling up the steps of public buildings on a regular basis. When they did, they participated in a masquerade for political ends. The network news cameras could not resist the sight of paraplegics dragging themselves up the Capitol steps. Some activists worried that the coverage pictured the image most people with disabilities want to avoid—that they are pitiable, weak, and childlike—and concluded that assuming this identity was not worth the publicity. Predictably, in fact, the cameras picked out exhausted, eight-year-old Jennifer Keelan for special attention, twisting the emphasis from the concerns of adults to those of children and suggesting that ADAPT was taking advantage of children for its cause. At the end of the day, however, the major networks stressed the important message that people with disabilities were demanding their civil rights.

The masquerade may serve as a form of communication, either between people sharing the same disability or as a message to able-bodied people that a disabled person is in their midst. "Stigma symbols have the character of being continuously available for perception," Goffman explains. "Fleeting offerings of evidence may be made—purposeful slips, as it were—as when a blind person voluntarily commits a clumsy act in the presence of newcomers as a way of informing them about his stigma" (101). Voluntary slips and disclosures always involve self-presentation, and when not an act of private communication between people with disabilities, they may serve a variety of purposes. They may send a sign to authority figures, who have a habit of swooping down violently without first asking questions, that the object of their attention requires a different mode of address. It is this strategy that tempts Joe Grigely when he ponders whether he should wear a red hearing aid to help manage the rudeness of people around him. Megan Jones details the strategy at greater length.[23] Legally blind and hearing impaired, she now uses a white cane in addition to a guide dog after having been assaulted many times by restaurant owners and other people for bringing her dog into forbidden places. Most people do not recognize her dog as a guide dog because of its breed, but the addition of the white cane allows her blindness and the use of her dog to register. Of course, such tactics do not always have the desired effect. Voluntary disclosure and exaggerated self-presentation may not be sufficient to render disability visible since the public is adept at ignoring people with disabilities. Authority figures will attack people for "faking" their disability, and if they are in fact exaggerating it, what stance can they take? The strategy is dangerous because it risks inflaming the anger of a public already irritated with disabled people.

   The masquerade may contravene an existing system of oppression. Reasons for the masquerade can be as simple as preserving energy and as complicated as making a joke or protest at the expense of the able-bodied. "Piqued at continuing to inconvenience myself," Irving Zola reports, "I began to regularly use a wheelchair" for excursions to the airport. "I thought that the only surprise I'd encounter would be the dubious glances of other passengers, when after reaching my destination, I would rise unassisted and walk briskly away."[24] Zola is able to make his way through the airport at the beginning and end of trips, but the overuse of energy may mean that he will not have enough strength later in the day or the next day to meet his obligations. He turns to the wheelchair because traveling requires overcompensation, and people with disabilities are never more disabled than when they are overcompensating. "Just because an individual *can* do something physical," Zola argues, "does not mean that he *should*" (Zola's italics, 232). The wheelchair allows him to claim disability, refusing both overcompensation and the ideological requirement that everyone be as able-bodied as possible.

   Airports and other public places unfriendly to people with disabilities also present a host of emotional obstacles in addition to physical ones. Zola mentions the "angry glances" of fellow travelers when he climbs staircases "too slowly" or impedes "the rush to seats on a bus" (209). As a person with a disability, he attracts the anger and hatred of people around him. He becomes their "cripple," a disdainful blemish on society and disruptive to the normal way of life. His disability is the cause of his inability to be part of society and its hatred of him. By using the wheelchair, he disrupts the cause-and-effect logic used to humiliate him on a daily basis. He discovers a creative solution, one that adjusts his needs to his environment and changes the psychology of the situation to his advantage. The masquerade, of course, does not necessarily change how people respond to him—he is now a wheelchair user getting in the way—but it does introduce a disruption in the causal logic of humiliation because Zola's identity is masked prophylactically and therefore unavailable to public disdain. He is not who they think he is. He is not where they think he is. He is a target on wheels.

The reverse side of the demand that disabled people overcompensate in public, both to meet the expectations of able-bodied people and to save them from inconvenience, is the masquerade. It meets the demand for overcompensation with undercompensation. Zola's use of the wheelchair improvises on his previous experience with the inaccessibility of public transportation and the reluctance of the general population to acknowledge the problem. His masquerade favors independence and self-preservation.

The masquerade may put expectations and prejudices about disability in the service of disabled people. Social prejudices about disability are rigid, and often people with disabilities are required to make their bodies conform to these expectations. As Goffman reports, the able-bodied "expect the cripple to be crippled; to be disabled and helpless: to be inferior to themselves, and they will become suspicious and insecure if the cripple falls short of these expectations" (110). Cal Montgomery provides examples of how actual behaviors contradict expectations about disability: "The person who uses a white cane when getting on the bus, but then pulls out a book to read while riding; the person who uses a wheelchair to get into the library stacks but then stands up to reach a book on a high shelf. . . . [T]he person who challenges the particular expectations of disability that other people have is suspect. 'I can't see what's wrong with him,' people say, meaning, 'He's not acting the way I think he should.'"[25] The masquerade may be used to expose false expectations, or it may use expectations to make life easier for the disabled person.

Prostheses play a crucial role in this process because they serve as indices of disability. Indexical signs, being denotative rather than connotative, point to other meanings, thereby summoning the array of representations signifying any given social practice or object of knowledge. These representations often have an ideological content, existing outside the awareness of society and supporting clichés and stereotypes. Montgomery captures the relation between disability and the indexical property of prostheses with great simplicity and vividness: "When nondisabled people look at 'the disabled,'" he explains, "they see wheelchairs and picture-boards. They see helmets and hearing aids and white canes. With a few exceptions, they don't pick up on how individuals differ from one another; they notice the tools we use. And these tools, to the general public, equal 'disability.' Venture out without a well-known tool, and your disability is 'invisible' or 'hidden.'"[26]

People with disabilities risk becoming their prostheses, Montgomery worries, and this symbolism is demoralizing. But it also provides a resource for changing the meaning of disability. On the one hand, prosthetics tends to establish a law of substitution, diverting attention away from the disabled organ to its replacement. Kenny Fries reports that his crippled legs attract more attention than those of a friend who uses crutches. "I have noticed," he writes, "that although he walks with crutches his legs do not call the same kind of attention to him as mine do, as if the crutches serve as a satisfying explanation for the different way he walks."[27] People in the street ask Fries what is wrong with him and ignore his companion, suggesting that uninvited stares are diverted to prostheses, absorbed there, and satisfied, while disabled limbs spark endless curiosity and anxiety. On the other hand, the powerful symbolic connection between disability and prosthetics allows those who improvise on the use of their prosthesis to tinker with the social meaning of their disability. Anne Finger recounts her experience with a new kind of motorized wheelchair, as yet unfamiliar to most passersby: "People were forever stopping me on the street and saying, 'What is that?' When I said, 'a wheelchair,' they would invariably smile very broadly, say, 'I'm sorry,' and move backwards."[28] The instant the new machine is named as a "wheelchair," it assumes its indexical quality as a sign of disability, and people, who moments before approached its user with a sense of curiosity, back away with a sense of dread.

Of course, Finger could have represented her wheelchair in a way resistant to prejudices about disability. In fact, users may work the meaning of their disability by using different applications of their prosthesis. Jaclyn Stuart switches between prosthetic hands, depending on the effect she wants to achieve. She wears a nonfunctional, rubber cosmetic hand to avoid stares of revulsion in some intimate public situations: "I wear it when I go dancing because otherwise [if I wear my hook] the whole dance floor goes crazy!" But she views her hook prosthesis as a symbol of liberation from normalization: "[W]hen I see the hook, I say, boy, what a *bad* broad. And that's the look I like best."[29] Wooden crutches rather than forearm crutches may allow their user to "fly under the radar," avoiding prejudices against people with long-term disabilities and assuming "visitor status" among the sick. People who require assistance walking participate at times in a complex semiotics of canes, using different types to mark themselves according to received ideas about age, gender, sex, and character types. The purposeful misapplication of prostheses introduces a temporary confusion in the public mind, allowing users a brief moment of freedom in which to assert their independence and individuality.

Many representations of people with disabilities, however, use narrative structures that masquerade disability for the benefit of the able-bodied public. Human-interest stories display voyeuristically the physical or mental disability of their heroes, making the defect emphatically present, often exaggerating it, and then wiping it away by reporting about how it has been overcome, how the heroes are "normal," despite the powerful odds against them. At other times, a story will work so hard to make its protagonist "normal" that it pictures the disabled person as possessing talents and abilities only dreamed about by able-bodied people. In other words, the hero is—simultaneously and incoherently—"cripple" and "supercripple." This image of disability belongs to the masquerade because it serves a larger ideology requiring the exaggeration of disability, although here it is for the benefit of the able-bodied audience, not the disabled heroes themselves, and this fact makes all the difference. Unlike the cases examined so far, this variety of the masquerade advantages able-bodied society more than disabled people because it affirms the ideology of able-bodiedness. This ideology represses disability by representing the able-body as the baseline in the definition of the human, and because human-interest stories usually require their hero to be human, they are obliged, when the focus is disability, to give an account of their protagonist's metamorphosis from nonhuman to human being.

Two typical human-interest stories about disabled heroes help to flesh out the ideology informing this type of masquerade. The first gives an account of Herbert M. Greenberg, blind since the age of ten, who founded a human-resources consulting firm, Caliper Management, that gives advice about the personality of job applicants to many famous companies, including the NBA.[30] A mutant strain of tuberculosis took Greenberg's sight in 1940. Public schools turned him away, and other boys beat him up at summer camp. But he was "motivated by adversity" and eventually earned a doctorate in social work from New York University. Nevertheless, most universities were not interested in hiring a blind professor, and after teaching stints in the '50s and '60s, while selling insurance on the side, he developed a psychological test that measures character traits like risk taking, empathy, and resilience. He started Caliper with an associate, and today having administered 1.8 million tests, the firm has a stable of loyal clients.

The first lines of the story connect Greenberg's blindness directly to his ability to assess job applicants fairly: "Blind people can't easily tell if a job candidate is white or black, thin or obese, plain or pretty. So if they should happen to assess an applicant's professional qualifications, they might well focus on a more mundane matter: Is she actually suited for the job?" As the figure of blind justice, Greenberg shows the ability, through his disability, to do what sighted people cannot: he is blind to the prejudices that bias judgment. The figure of the blind judge, however, is merely a trope because it purposefully represses facts about blindness as well as about Greenberg's actual role in the narrative. On the one hand, the story misrepresents blindness as if it blocked all sensory perception. Sight loss, however, exists in different ranges, and blind people can gather a great deal of information about the people around them. Senses other than sight also provide information about the physical, gender, and racial characteristics of people. The story masquerades Greenberg as blinder than he is in order to establish him as the epitome of impartial judgment. On the other hand, Greenberg's other talents, ones able-bodied people do not always possess, make up for his blindness. The story must confirm that he has abilities that compensate for his disability if it is to privilege ability over disability as the ideological baseline of humanness. Despite his blindness, then, Greenberg is supposedly more perceptive than other people. John Gabriel, general manager of the Orlando Magic, introduces this idea when praising the scouting advice of his "blind consultant": "Sometimes analyzing a player involves what you can't see, the intangibles. They may be heart, hustle, drive, determination, leadership. Herb Greenberg can identify those for you."[31] Of course, the fact that Greenberg assesses applicants by psychological test and not personal interview is ignored in order to establish the trope of the totally blind judge who nevertheless has extraordinary powers of perception about the moral and psychological character of other human beings. The story creates a persona for its protagonist that masquerades what disability is.

The second example is a human-interest story recounting the remarkable artistic success, "despite autism," of Jonathan Lerman, a fourteen-year-old charcoal artist, "retarded with an I.Q. of 53," who began to draw at age ten "in the way of savants."[32] His specialty is portraits, although "most autistic artists don't show faces." Moreover, one authority has compared the work favorably to portraits by George Grosz and Francis Bacon, "without the horror and shame." "Raising him was heartbreaking," his mother reports, because of his uncontrollable and baffling behavior. At the lakeside he stepped on the bodies of sunbathers, as if they were part of the beach; he took food from other people's plates at restaurants without asking; and he refused to eat pizza with oregano and cheese bubbles. His artistic gifts are equally puzzling, the story continues, since "science is still struggling to understand what two Harvard neurologists have called 'the pathology of superiority,' the linkage of gift and disorder that explains how someone unable to communicate or perform simple tasks can at the same time calculate astronomical sums or produce striking music or art." In short, Lerman's disability and ability, the story asks the reader to believe, are well beyond the normal range of experience.

The general, descriptive phrase, "pathology of superiority," sums up nicely the paradox of human-interest stories about disability. The obligatory shift from disability to superability that characterizes the stories serves to conflate pathology with claims of exceptional talent. Each sentence in the story about Lerman carries the burden of this paradox. Here is, for example, an apparently simple and straightforward portrait of the artist as a young man with a disability. "Flowing from Jonathan's clutched charcoal, five and ten sheets at a sitting, came faces of throbbing immediacy, harrowing and comical."[33] Lerman cannot hold his charcoal but clutches it. His works of art seem to flow not from his talent but from his disability. Words like "clutched" and "throbbing" lend pathology to his behavior, contaminating the more familiar language about artistic inspiration and talent. His ability is rendered dubious as a result, but not less dubious than his disability, because both rely on the masquerade.

Not surprisingly, what distinguishes Lerman's drawings from other works of art is what attracts and disturbs art lovers the most. The portraits, like many examples of art brut, are "uncooked by cultural influences."[34] They pass the test of originality because they diverge from cliché, but since their origin is unfathomable, they also seem unnerving. John Thomson, chairman of the art department at Binghamton University, captures succinctly the contradictory impulse that this story attaches to Lerman—an impulse that marks him simultaneously as normal and abnormal. His work "would not be out of place in my classroom," Thomson explains, but it is also "really exceptional, characterized by an amazing lack of stereotypes common to drawings at all age levels." Similarly, the story takes pains to tell its readers that one of Lerman's idols is rock star Kurt Cobain, that his drawings are beginning to include references to sex and MTV, while stressing repeatedly how far removed he is from normal society. The punch line describes the young artist's happiness, despite his supposedly diminished capacity to be happy, with the fact that people love his art, suggesting some kind of breakthrough produced by his artistic abilities: "To what extent Jonathan knows the hit he has made is not clear. 'Jonathan's capacity to understand is not that great,' Mrs. Lerman said. 'I said, "People really love your art," and he was happy.'"

Human-interest stories do not focus as a rule on people with disabilities who fail to show some extraordinary ability. Blind women who run at Olympic pace, talented jazz musicians with Tourette's syndrome, deaf heart surgeons, or famous actors with a stutter are the usual stuff of these narratives. In each case, ability trumps disability, creating a morality tale about one person's journey from disease to cure, from inhumanity to humanity. These accounts fit with the masquerade because they exaggerate the disability of their heroes, suggesting that it is a mask that can be easily removed to uncover the real human being beneath. But they also exaggerate in the process the connection between able-bodiedness and humanness, giving happy relief and assurance to those who consider themselves healthy.

Imagine if health were really the hallmark of one's humanity, if it were in fact possible to go through life without ever being sick. The result would be unbelievable and undesirable, and yet it is exactly what many stories about disability ask us to believe and to desire: "What would it be like for [a] person to go through life never being sick?" Anne Finger asks. "A man or woman of steel, a body impervious to disease, never facing those deaths of the old physical self that are a sort of skin-shedding" (43).

A final variety of the masquerade, related to the type informing human-interest stories about people with disabilities, I call "disability drag." It, too, represses disability. Drag, of course, lines up oddly with passing, but the masquerade does as well, so it may be productive to consider the masquerade in the light of drag. The best cases of disability drag are found in those films in which an able-bodied actor plays disabled. I make reference to drag because the performance of the able-bodied actor is usually as bombastic as a drag performance. Esther Newton argues that drag queens represent the "stigma of the gay world" because they make the stigma most visible (3). While there are certain people with disabilities who embody the stigma of disability more visibly than others—and the masquerade permits the exaggeration of disability by people with disabilities—the most obvious markings of disability as a spoiled identity occur in the performances of able-bodied actors. The modern cinema often puts the stigma of disability on display, except that films exhibit the stigma not to insiders by insiders, as is the usual case with drag, but to a general public that does not realize it is attending a drag performance. In short, when we view an able-bodied actor playing disabled, we have the same experience of exaggeration and performance as when we view a man playing a woman.[35] Audiences, however, rarely recognize the symmetry. Dustin Hoffman does not pass as a woman in *Tootsie* (1982). Nor does he pass as disabled in *Rain Man* (1988). Audiences nevertheless have entirely different reactions to the two performances—they know the first performance is a fake but accept the second one as Oscar worthy—and yet Hoffman's performance in *Rain Man* is as much a drag performance as his work in *Tootsie*. In fact, the narrative structures of the two films are the same. In *Rain Man*, Hoffman's character, Raymond, may be an autistic savant, but it is his brother Charlie who cannot relate to other people. Among Raymond's many gifts is his ability to pull Charlie out of his "autism" and teach him how to love and trust other people. Similarly, Hoffman's character in *Tootsie* puts himself in touch with his feminine side by doing drag, but his real accomplishment is to teach the women of America to stand up for themselves and to embrace their femininity as a strength, not a disability.

I Am Sam (2002) provides another more recent use of disability drag. Some critics have praised the film as an accurate representation of "mental retardation." It has actors with disabilities in supporting roles, including one with Down's syndrome. Sean Penn, however, plays Sam, a man with the intelligence of a seven-year-old trying to retain custody of his seven-year-old, able-bodied daughter, Lucy. Regardless of the power of his Oscar-nominated performance, it is difficult to agree that the film portrays disability accurately because accuracy does not lie only in the performance of actors but in the overall narrative structure and plot of films, and here the film fails miserably. Its use of music as a commentary on disability stigmatizes Sam, and the film creates scene after scene designed to set him apart as a freak. The final scene is paradigmatic of how the film treats him. It is a happy and triumphant scene staged at a soccer game at which the community is celebrating the fact that Sam has finally won custody of Lucy. Incomprehensibly, Sam appears as the referee of the soccer match. This plot twist places him in the action of the game but magnifies his disability by contrasting it with the duties usually performed by a referee. Instead of officiating the game and striving to be neutral in his calls, he cheers on Lucy, pursuing her all over the field, and when she scores a goal, he lifts her into his arms and runs in giddy circles, while an excited troop of children chase him and the adults whoop and cheer on the sidelines.

The advantage of disability drag is that it prompts audiences to embrace disability. Its disadvantage is that disability appears as a facade overlaying able-bodiedness. The use of able-bodied actors, whose bombastic performances represent their able-bodiedness as much as their pretence of disability, not only keeps disability out of public view but transforms its reality and its fundamental characteristics. It renders disability invisible because able-bodied people substitute for people with disabilities, similar to white performers who put on blackface at minstrel shows or to straight actors who play "fag" to bad comic effect. As a result, the audience perceives the disabled body as a sign of the acting abilities of the performer—the more disabled the character, the greater the ability of the actor. Disability drag also transforms disability by insinuating ability into its reality and representation. When actors play disabled in one film and able-bodied in the next, the evolution of the roles presents them as cured of a previous disease or condition. The audience also knows that an actor will return to an able-bodied state as soon as the film ends.[36] Disability drag is a variety of the masquerade, then, providing an exaggerated exhibition of people with disabilities but questioning both the existence and permanence of disability. It acts as a lure for the fantasies and fears of able-bodied audiences and reassures them that the threat of disability is not real, that everything was only pretend—unlike the masquerade used by people with disabilities, where the mask, once removed, reveals the reality and depth of disability existing beneath it.

IV.

Disability activists are fond of pointing out that there are a thousand ways to be disabled but that able-bodied people are all alike.

This is true only metaphorically, of course, since variation thrives in every facet of human existence, but it is worth emphasizing because the ideology of able-bodiedness makes a powerful call on everyone in society to embrace uniformity. The desire to pass is a symptom of this call. The hope of those who try to pass is that no one will have anything different to say about them. Passing compels one to blend in, to be the same, to be normal. Barry Adam asserts that passing supports the "general inequality" of society with the promise of opportunity but benefits very few people in the final analysis.[37] Those who pass improve their own life, but they fail to change the existing system of social privilege and economic distribution. They may win greater acceptance and wealth but only by pretending to be someone they are not and supporting the continued oppression of the group to which they do belong.

The masquerade counteracts passing, claiming disability rather than concealing it. Exaggerating or performing difference, when that difference is a stigma, marks one as a target, but it also exposes and resists the prejudices of society. The masquerade fulfills a desire to tell a story about disability, often the very story that society does not want to hear because it refuses to obey the ideology of able-bodiedness. It may stress undercompensation when overcompensation is required, or present a coming out of disability when invisibility is mandatory. As a consequence, the masquerade produces what Adam calls "overvisibility," a term of disparagement aimed at minority groups who appear to be "too much" for society to bear but also a phenomenon that nevertheless carries potential for political action (49). Women who make demands on men are "too pushy." African Americans are "too boisterous" and "too noisy" around white people. Gay men are "too flashy" and "too effeminate" for straight taste. People with disabilities should stay out of sight because able-bodied society finds them "too ugly." Overstated differences and feigned disabilities serve as small conspiracies against oppression and inequality. They subvert existing social conventions, and they contribute to the solidarity of marginal groups by seizing control of stereotypes and resisting the pressure to embrace norms of behavior and appearance.

The masquerade exists in two perspectives, the point of view of the disabled and the nondisabled. The first tells a story to the second, but each side expresses a desire, the desire to see disability as other than it is. The question is whether it is the same desire on both sides, whether there are resources for interfering with the desire to pass, whether other stories exist. The masquerade presents us with the opportunity to explore alternative narratives, to ask what happens when disability is claimed as some version of itself rather than simply concealed from view.

NOTES

1. On the rhetoric of coming out as a person with a disability, see Brenda Jo Brueggemann, "'It's So Hard to Believe That You Pass': A Hearing-Impaired Student Writing on the Borders of Language" and "On (Almost) Passing," in *Lend Me Your Ear: Rhetorical Constructions of Deafness* (Washington, DC: Gallaudet University Press, 1999), 50–80, 81–99; Brenda Jo Brueggemann and Georgina Kleege, "Gently Down the Stream: Reflections on Mainstreaming," *Rhetoric Review* 22, no. 2 (2003): 174–84; Georgina Kleege, "Disabled Students Come Out: Questions without Answers," in *Disability Studies: Enabling the Humanities,* ed. Sharon L. Snyder, Brenda Jo Brueggemann, and Rosemarie Garland-Thomson (New York: MLA, 2002) , 308–16; Rod Michalko, *The Mystery of the Eye and the Shadow of Blindness* (Toronto: University of Toronto Press, 1998); and Mitchell Tepper, "Coming Out as a Person with a Disability," *Disability Studies Quarterly* 19, no. 2 (1999): 105–6. On the limits of coming-out discourse, see Ellen Jean Samuels, "My Body, My Closet: Invisible Disability and the Limits of Coming-Out Discourse," *GLQ* 9, no. 1–2 (2003): 233–55.

2. Erving Goffman, *Stigma: Notes on the Management of Spoiled Identity* (Englewood Cliffs, NJ: Prentice-Hall, 1963). Subsequent references are cited parenthetically in the text.

3. Eve Kosofsky Sedgwick, *Epistemology of the Closet* (Berkeley: University of California Press, 1990), 72. Subsequent references are cited parenthetically in the text.

4. Linda Greenhouse, "High Court Limits Who is Protected by Disability Law," *New York Times,* June 23, 1999, A1, A16.

5. See Janet E. Halley, *Don't: A Reader's Guide to the Military's Anti-Gay Policy* (Durham, NC: Duke University Press, 1999).

6. Patricia J. Williams, *The Alchemy of Race and Rights* (Cambridge: Harvard University Press, 1991), 213–36. Williams theorizes staring, playing on the difference between being visible and being recognized. She notes that as a black woman she is highly marked and socially invisible at the same time. In fact, it is the heightened visibility of her blackness that produces her social invisibility.

7. See also Esther Newton, *Mother Camp: Female Impersonators in America* (Chicago: University of Chicago Press, 1979). Newton provides a counterexample, explaining that drag queens represent the shame of the gay world because they most visibly embody the stigma (3). Subsequent references are cited parenthetically in the text.

8. Barbara Christian, "The Race for Theory," in *The Nature and Context of Minority Discourse,* ed. Abdul R. JanMohamed and David Lloyd (New York: Oxford University Press, 1990), 37–49. The essays in María Carla Sánchez and Linda Schlossberg, eds., *Passing: Identity and Interpretation in Sexuality, Race, and Religion* (New York: New York University Press, 2001) discuss passing as a method of establishing alternative narratives. Judith Butler is also important to the theory of passing. For consideration of her work in the context of disability studies, see Ellen Jean Samuels, "Critical Divides: Judith Butler's Body Theory and the Question of Disability," *NWSA Journal* 14, no. 3 (2002): 58–76; Tobin Siebers, "Disability in Theory: From Social Construction to the New Realism of the Body," *American Literary History* 13, no. 4 (2001): 737–54; and Siebers, "Disability and the Future of Identity Politics," in *Redefining Identity Politics,* ed. Linda Martín Alcoff, Satya Mohanty, and Paula Moya (New York: Palgrave-MacMillan, forthcoming). See Judith Butler, *Gender Trouble:*

Feminism and the Subversion of Identity (New York: Routledge, 1999) and *Bodies That Matter: On the Discursive Limits of "Sex"* (New York: Routledge, 1993).

9. Joan Riviere, "Womanliness as a Masquerade," in *The Inner World and Joan Riviere: Collected Papers: 1920–1958*, ed. Athol Hughes (London: Karnac Books, 1991), 90–101, originally published in the *International Journal of Psycho-Analysis* 9 (1929): 303–13. Subsequent references are cited parenthetically in the text.

10. A good introduction to the complexities of racial passing is Adrian Piper, "Passing for White, Passing for Black," *Transition* 58 (1992): 4–32, 18. For other important treatments of racial passing, see Deborah E. McDowell, introduction to *Quicksand and Passing*, by Nella Larson (New Brunswick, NJ: Rutgers University Press, 1986); Phillip Brian Harper, "Gender Politics and the 'Passing' Fancy: Black Masculinity as Societal Problem," in *Are We Not Men? Masculine Anxiety and the Problem of African-American Identity* (New York: Oxford University Press, 1996), 103–26; Robyn Wiegman, *American Anatomies: Theorizing Race and Gender* (Durham, NC: Duke University Press, 1995); Werner Sollors, *Neither Black Nor White Yet Both: Thematic Explorations of Interracial Literature* (New York: Oxford University Press, 1997); Richard Dyer, "White," *Screen* 29, no. 4 (1988): 44–64; and Gayle Wald, *Crossing the Line: Racial Passing in Twentieth-Century U.S. Literature and Culture* (Durham, NC: Duke University Press, 2000). It is worth mentioning that the idea of achieving "color-blind" or "race-blind" societies needs someday to be interrogated from a disability perspective alert to the metaphor of blindness.

11. A number of theorists have described the masquerade as a strategy that manages stigma by creating effects subversive to male power. See Mary Ann Doane, "Film and the Masquerade: Theorising the Female Spectator," *Screen* 23, no. 3–4 (1982): 74–87 and its sequel, "Masquerade Reconsidered: Further Thoughts on the Female Spectator," *Discourse* 11 (1988–9): 42–54; Teresa de Lauretis, "Feminist Studies/Critical Studies: Issues, Terms, and Contexts," in *Feminist Studies, Critical Studies*, ed. Teresa de Lauretis (Bloomington: Indiana University Press, 1986), 1–19, esp. 17; Terry Castle, *Masquerade and Civilization: The Carnivalesque in Eighteenth-Century English Culture and Fiction* (Stanford, CA: Stanford University Press, 1986); and Marjorie Garber, *Vested Interests: Cross-Dressing and Cultural Anxiety* (New York: Routledge, 1992), esp. 10.

12. Joseph Grigely, "Postcards to Sophie Calle," in *The Body Aesthetic: From Fine Art to Body Modification*, ed. Tobin Siebers (Ann Arbor: University of Michigan Press, 2000), 17–40, 28.

13. See Adrienne Rich, "Compulsory Heterosexuality and Lesbian Existence," in *Women: Sex and Sexuality*, ed. Catharine R. Stimpson and Ethel Spector Person (Chicago: University of Chicago Press, 1980), 62–91; and Robert McRuer, "Compulsory Able-Bodiedness and Queer/Disabled Existence," in Snyder et al., *Disability Studies: Enabling the Humanities*, 88–99.

14. Of course, Riviere may be masquerading herself. See Stephen Heath, "Joan Riviere and the Masquerade," in *Formations of Fantasy*, ed. Victor Burgin, James Donald, and Cora Kaplan (London: Methuen, 1986), 45–61.

15. See Sigmund Freud, "Some Character-Types Met with in Psycho-Analytic Work," in *The Standard Edition*, ed. and trans. James Strachey (London: Hogarth, 1953–74), 14: 309–33, esp. 315.

16. See Harold Bloom, *The Western Canon: The Books and School of the Ages* (New York: Harcourt Brace and Company, 1994); and Wendy Brown, *States of Injury: Power and Freedom in Late Modernity* (Princeton, NJ: Princeton University Press, 1995).

17. Stephen Heath prefers a political reading as well. He argues that the woman "puts on a show of the femininity" demanded by her male colleagues as a "charade of power" designed to meet masculine authority with its own fantasies and fears of woman (56). He places the masquerade not in the context of sadism and rivalry but in the context of "sexual politics" and "protest" (56).

18. See Tom Shakespeare, "Disability, Identity, Difference," in *Exploring the Divide: Illness and Disability*, ed. Colin Barnes and Geof Mercer (Leeds: Disability Press, 1996), 94–113, esp. 100; Simi Linton, *Claiming Disability: Knowledge and Identity* (New York: New York University Press, 1998); and Robert McRuer, "As Good as It Gets: Queer Theory and Critical Disability," *GLQ* 9, no. 1–2 (2003): 79–105.

19. On the theoretical value of identity, see Tobin Siebers, *Morals and Stories* (New York: Columbia University Press, 1992), esp. chaps. 2 and 4.

20. On the use of disability identity to illuminate the social construction of reality, see Tobin Siebers, "Disability and the Future of Identity Politics" and "Social Facts: One or Two Things We Know about Disability," paper, "Redefining Identity Politics: Internationalism, Feminism, Multiculturalism," University of Michigan, Ann Arbor, MI, October 18, 2002.

21. Paula M. L. Moya, *Learning from Experience: Minority Identities, Multicultural Struggles* (Berkeley: University of California Press, 2002), 27 (Moya's italics).

22. For an account of the protest events, see Joseph Shapiro, *No Pity: People with Disabilities Forging a New Civil Rights Movement* (New York: Three Rivers Press, 1993), 131–41.

23. Megan Jones, "'Gee, You Don't *Look* Handicapped . . .' Why I Use a White Cane to Tell People I'm Deaf," *Electric Edge* (July/August 1997), http://www.ragged-edge-mag.com/archive/look.htm (accessed March 18, 2004).

24. Irving Zola, *Missing Pieces: A Chronicle of Living with a Disability* (Philadelphia: Temple University Press, 1982), 205. Subsequent references are cited parenthetically in the text.

25. References are to Cal Montgomery, "A Hard Look at Invisible Disability," *Ragged Edge Magazine Online* 2 (2001), http://www.ragged-edge-mag.com/0301/0301ft1.htm (accessed on March 17, 2004).

26. Ibid.

27. Kenny Fries, *Body, Remember: A Memoir* (New York: Blume, 1998), 110.

28. Anne Finger, *Past Due: A Story of Disability, Pregnancy and Birth* (Seattle, WA: Seal Press, 1990), 26. Subsequent references are cited parenthetically in the text.

29. Cited by Marilynn J. Phillips, "Damaged Goods: Oral Narratives of the Experience of Disability in American Culture," *Social Science and Medicine* 30, no. 8 (1990): 849–57, 855 (Phillips's italics).

30. References are to Geoffrey Brewer, "Oh, the Psyches and Personalities He Has Seen," *New York Times*, April 19, 2000, C10.

31. Ibid.

32. References are to Ralph Blumenthal, "An Artist's Success at 14, Despite Autism," *New York Times*, January 16, 2002, E1.

33. Ibid.

34. Ibid.

35. Disability drag also invites connections to drag kinging. See Judith Halberstam, *Female Masculinity* (Durham, NC: Duke University Press, 1998), 231–66, and "Oh Behave! Austin Powers and the Drag Kings," *GLQ* 7, no. 3 (2001): 425–52, esp. 427.

36. Deborah Marks, *Disability: Controversial Debates and Psychosocial Perspectives* (London: Routledge, 1999), 160, suggests that the real reason for using nondisabled actors for disabled parts is to reassure the audience that disability is not real.

37. Barry D. Adam, *The Survival of Domination: Inferiorization and Everyday Life* (New York: Elsevier, 1978), 119. Subsequent references are cited parenthetically in the text.

Meditation, Disability, and Identity

Susan Squier

> Since we are all Crips in one way or another, it is well worth learning the truth of what must befall us some day, even if it hasn't already started (it has).
>
> Lorenzo Milam, *CripZen: A Manual for Survival*

> After all, when all identities are finally included, there will be no identity.
>
> Lennard Davis, *Bending Over Backwards*

> [C]lassifications should be recognized as the significant site of political and ethical work that they are. They should be reclassified. . . . There is no simple unraveling of the built information landscape, or, *pace* Zen practice, of unsettling our habits at every waking moment.
>
> Bowker and Star, *Sorting Things Out*

I have practiced Zen meditation for a number of years now. Maybe that is why, when I noticed that a number of disabled people have taken up meditation and written narratives about it, I became interested in what meditation has to teach us about disability (and vice-versa). Seated meditation, or *zazen*, involves learning to "think not-thinking," according to Zen Master Dogen.[1] Zazen consists of the moment-to-moment encounter with *what is*: the thoughts that flow through the mind; the feelings that pass through the body; and the occurrences in one's surroundings as they come into being, and fade away.

An examination of three narratives written by disabled meditators reveals how Zen meditation might illuminate the relationship between disability and identity, as well as what Buddhism might learn from the experience of disability. Lorenzo Milam writes *CripZen: A Manual for Survival* from the perspective of a postpolio paraplegic.[2] Joan Tollifson, whose right hand was severed in utero by a strand of amniotic tissue, traces her journey from alienated marginality through disability activism to committed meditation practitioner in her *Bare-Bones Meditation*.[3] Finally, in *The Zen Path through Depression,* Philip Martin investigates the value of meditation to a social worker and psychotherapist suffering from major depression, a disability generally situated on the other side of the mind/body divide from the experiences of Milam and Tollifson.[4] In these three narratives, Zen insight is modified by disability insight, so that meditation acts as a survival aid for the disabled person at the same time as the experience of disability modifies the notion of meditation, introducing itself as a new form of Zen practice. But what of narratives written not by disabled meditators, but by those who treat the disabled? If we examine two recent studies by medical and psychological professionals who use meditation as a mode of treatment, we can see that the two-way traffic between meditation and disability is given another twist in clinical texts written from the point of view of the practitioner.[5] As I will explore, the result is a paradoxical identity position with challenging implications for disability studies.

Milam, Tollifson, and Martin arguably have very different experiences of body and mind, given their very different disabilities, but through meditation they learn the inadequacy of any simple construction of the disabled identity, whether universalizing or minoritizing.[6] To frame a universalizing view of disability would be to say, with Lennard Davis, "People with disability: they are you."[7] Such a view extends disability from a narrow category of difference to a broad category with, sooner or later, universal applicability. Viewed this way, the identity category of disability is porous; as it reconceptualizes ability, it decenters the norm. Philosopher Eva Kittay makes strategic use of this position when she argues that disability is characterized by the dependency that all human beings share at least twice in our lives: when we are infants, and when we are very old.[8] The minoritizing view retains the concept of "normal" and holds that only the person with a disability has the right to represent the disabled. As James Charlton puts it in his study of disability-rights activists around the world, "This is a militant, revelational claim aptly capsulized in 'Nothing About Us Without Us.'"[9] The slogan asserts marginality in order to claim representation as disabled Others, a strategy distinct (in philosophy and in historical use) from the universalizing claim that disability is an inevitable life experience.[10]

These narratives by disabled meditators point to an epistemological or representational gap between the embrace of disability as a collective constructed identity and the Zen-influenced surrender of any notion of identity at all. This gap is reflected in the uncertain genre of these texts, all of which offer what might be called the "situated knowledges" made possible by meditating with a disability. This term, which has a Zen-like paradox at its core, I draw from Donna Haraway, who describes it as "an ungraspable middle space": "even the simplest matters in feminist analysis require contradictory moments and a wariness of their resolution, dialectically or otherwise. 'Situated knowledges' is a shorthand term for this insistence."[11]

Lorenzo Milam's *CripZen:* A Manual for Survival

Lorenzo Milam contracted polio in 1952, as an eighteen-year-old Yale undergraduate. His dazzling, angry memoir, *The Cripple Liberation Front Marching Band Blues* (1984), recounts how he fell ill with polio just two weeks after his twenty-nine-year-old sister did.[12] (She would soon die of the disease.) A pioneer organizer of nonprofit radio stations, Milam wrote the classic handbook, *The Original Sex and Broadcasting: A Handbook on Starting a Radio Station for the Community*. Under the pseudonym Carlos Amantea he published *The Blob That Ate Oaxaca*, which was nominated for the Pulitzer Prize in 1992, while as "Pastor A. W. Allworthy," he investigated the tensions between the views on disability articulated in the Bible and Zen Buddhism. Milam abandoned the play with alternate identities in *CripZen*, however, which was published under his own name in 1993. He gave it the subtitle *A Manual for Survival* and addressed it to "those of us who have lost the use of part or all of our bodies. . . . With or without a label," he says, "we know who we are" (vii).

A compilation of pieces Milam wrote when he was "disability-sexuality columnist" for *Independent Living*, articles for other disability periodicals, reviews, and National Public Radio broadcasts, *CripZen* offers its readers a way of getting free "of the prisons: those we build for ourselves, and those created by people trying to help us" (171). Milam introduces the reader to a range of strategies including psychotherapy, hallucinogens, yoga, forms of sexuality ranging from sex surrogacy and masturbation to celibacy, and, in the title chapter, training in Zen meditation. All of these methods spring from what Milam calls his "two articles of faith." The first article is that each person with a disability will one day experience not just the revelation of "our new life" as disabled people, but what he calls the "Second Revelation": the realization that "our great bravery, our seeming acceptance of fate, the splendid triumph of spirit over physical self—these were all put-up jobs" (x). Milam explains that the pain of this discovery is almost overwhelming: "Once we come to the knowledge of the deception we have imposed on ourselves and on others, we find ourselves immersed in a new pain, and a bitter, bitter sadness. This can be fatal, as fatal as our first grief-at-loss" (xi). Milam suggests that the Second Revelation is responsible for the "possible fifty percent suicide rate" among "Crips. You and me" (ix). To combat that threat, Milam responds with mordant humor by modifying Kubler-Ross's five stages of dying to produce "five stages leading to CripZen":

> Stage I. I am not a Crip;
> Stage II. I'm a Crip, and I can't take it;
> Stage III. I'm a Crip, but I can beat it;
> Stage IV. I'm a Crip, I can beat it—but I am Still a Crip and
> I can't take it;
> Stage V. I am that I am. (223)[13]

"How to get from I to V without going under is the subject of this book," he explains (xii). That the Second Revelation "doesn't have to kill you," Milam offers as his "second article of faith." "Once you stumble across the truth of your being, . . . [it] will become part of your survival mechanism, one that even *you* won't be able to take from you. With it you can forge a powerful new system for dealing with a new world" (xi, Milam's italics).

CripZen does more than explore what meditation can do for the disabled; it demonstrates what disability consciousness can do for meditation, and then it goes beyond that to demonstrate the limitations of both. While his CripZen dharma recalls the traditional, repetitive, oral form of Buddhist sutras, it also subverts the authority of traditional Buddhism, challenging its normalizing foundations. Milam critiques Buddhist teachings for their ableist assumptions: "Some masters tell us that we can only do meditation in the lotus position. Obviously, they haven't gone through Rehab." With his ironic refrain, "You and I might be in an especially good position to study this," he asserts that the disabled meditator holds a privileged position as dharma student (192).

Milam's survival guide for the new world of disability has a central paradox: it simultaneously celebrates and relinquishes the body, mourning and embracing the disablement that is central to its loss. As he explains in the book's preface: "I must accept reluctant responsibility for the contradiction of *CripZen*—that is, that I offer a plea for Good Sex and Good Mental Health while at the same time offering a Zen model of Forget-The-Body Quiet-The-Mind" (viii). Notice the two-way traffic here. Zen meditation modifies the experience of disability, while disability modifies Zen practice.

While the book's title chapter opens with the assertion that "CripZen begins the day you wake up and know that you no longer own your body," Milam is far from arguing that when disablement occurs the longing for an able body has vanished, or even *should vanish* (171). Rather, Milam harnesses the paradoxical perspective of Zen doctrine to the goal of disability equity, offering in the concluding chapter a comic vision of the embodiment he would choose if he were reincarnated:

> I would still like to have the chance to work out with someone else's body for a change. Jane Fonda's, say. . . . Or the dusky, sunny fisher-lad we saw . . . in Puerto Perdido. . . . The one with the great sloe eyes, and the body like chocolate glacé, and the great quadriceps. . . . If they want me to come back with any real enthusiasm they'll have to stuff me into a body like that . . . I simply refuse to come back as a Crip gringo anymore, with all that dysfunctional plumbing, arms and legs that don't work worth shit, ridiculous aches and pains that take up too much of my days and nights. (250)

Milam imagines persuading the divine powers to give him a beautifully functioning body by promising that he will "give up everything when I get through with the usual teen-age indiscretions. After just a few short years, I'll become a holy man, a wandering saddhu."[14] To some readers of this essay, Milam's articulation of the yearning for a nondisabled body suggests that he is stuck at stage four of the five stages leading to CripZen: "I'm a Crip, I can beat it—but I am Still a Crip and I can't take it." Yet I read this somewhat differently. Milam's text both challenges and affirms the meditation-born insight that we truly do not own or control our own body. Whether we are disabled or able, the physical pleasures of our existence are transient, with pain being a recurrent, inevitable reality. Milam makes the universality of this Zen insight explicit in a footnote: "It's a Western concept that we can wage a war with the body and—with sufficient determination—win. The truth is that none of us can triumph in a battle with our own mind, body, or soul" (x). In fact, the very notion of life as an attempt to *triumph* over the mind, body, or soul is beside the point, as absurd as the advertising slogan I have taped to my file cabinet: "In 28 minutes you'll be meditating like a zen monk!" Time is not our enemy, but the very condition of our being, to be accepted, even celebrated.

Joan Tollifson's *Bare-Bones Meditation*

The power of meditation as an alternative to doing battle with the body or the mind is also central to the disability narrative of Joan Tollifson. Born without a hand, Tollifson grew up with a sense of herself as damaged, a construction of her identity reinforced by physicians, family, and strangers alike. Right after her birth, her doctors engaged in a curious performance:

> Newborn, I was brought to a room where there was a large pillow. My father was called out of the waiting area and taken to this room by the doctor. My father was left alone in there with me and the large pillow. He understood finally that he was being given the chance to smother me. But he didn't do it.
> The doctor knocked. "Are you finished yet?" (1)

As a child, she says, she felt like "a kind of oxymoron. Sometimes strangers on the street would tell my mother that we were being punished by God. . . . The central theme of my life was thus in place early: I was different, asymmetrical, imperfect, special. . . . When I was very small and first heard about death, I dreamed recurrently about a person whose arm fell off, then the other arm, then each leg, until nothing was left. I was already on my way toward this mysterious disappearance" (2). Starting with that core sense of herself as imperfect but "special," Tollifson gradually took on other identifications: as lesbian, as alcoholic, and finally as disability activist, one of over a hundred people who in 1977 occupied the San Francisco Federal Building for a month in support of civil rights for the disabled. The experience taught her that, "In the same way that gay people automatically understand that gender roles are mostly an arbitrary construction, disabled people automatically understand something about the illusory nature of our attachment to the body, and our ideas about what's normal" (21). After the Federal Building occupation ended, Tollifson found a copy of Shunryu Suzuki's classic, *Zen Mind, Beginner's Mind,* and began to meditate, an experience that confirmed the way she had already come to understand her identity, as that of a disabled person. As she explains, her childhood dream of the person losing body parts, working her way "toward this mysterious disappearance," anticipated the encounter with "no-self" that is central to Zen practice.

Yet Tollifson's experiences as a disability activist and a lesbian woman made this kind of surrender of self (and of the fantasized control over the self) problematic, for reasons she was helped to understand by Mel Weitsman, abbot and teacher of the Berkeley Zen Center: "He said that Zen practice is perhaps particularly challenging and difficult for people like blacks or gays who are working on finding their identity in a certain sense, or regaining it, because this practice is about having no identity at all" (90). Moving beyond static categories, the practitioner of meditation encounters a time that is no time (and all time), a self that is no self (and all selves), and a space that is both no space and unlimited space. The very concept of identity, as the embodied union of a finite discrete mind and a finite discrete body, is revealed as an inadequate model for the richly complex perspective and experience meditation brings into being. In her memoir, Tollifson articulates this transformed understanding of identity in a way that reflects the influence of her teacher, Toni Packer, who after studying with Roshi Philip Kapleau at the Rochester Zen Center eventually abandoned the formal trappings of Zen practice, stripping meditation down to its bare bones. Packer's modification of Buddhist dharma converges productively with Tollifson's own phenomenological understanding of physical disability in a metaphor at once whimsical and ironic. Tollifson explains:

> Toni's work is like realizing that we're all put here in various bizarre costumes: black skin, white skin, amputations, old age, cerebral palsy, Down's syndrome. Some people get more bizarre costumes than others, but everyone gets one, without exception. And then no one really sees anyone else. We see the costume. We can't get past it. Some people never even realize they're at a costume party. (91)

Tollifson explains how her metaphor of life as a costume party articulates the reconfigured notion of identity as "no-self" that Zen meditation teaches:

> I experience myself as a regular person who happens to be wearing this strange costume without a right hand. (A friend of mine in California calls her German shepherd the one in the dog suit, and that's sort of how I feel, like the one in the amputee suit.) (91)[15]

Tollifson's metaphor not only builds on Packer's work as a meditation teacher but critiques it as well, talking back to Buddhism by challenging what lies beneath the metaphor of life as a costume party. Her image offers a disability-based reformulation of the Zen practice of no-self, by revealing the unexamined *normate* assumptions of Zen doctrine. The term is Rosemarie Garland-Thomson's, and it refers to "the constructed identity of those who, by way of the bodily configurations and cultural capital they assume, can step into a position of authority and wield the power it grants them."[16]

Garland-Thomson connects the binary oppositions that structure normate and non-normate identities to the binary oppositions unhelpfully structuring homo/heterosexual identities: "Naming the figure of the normate is one conceptual strategy that will allow us to press our analyses beyond the simple dichotomies of male/female, white/black, straight/gay, or able-bodied/disabled so that we can examine the subtle interrelations among social identities that are anchored to physical differences."[17] While meditation may afford the valuable insight that we're "all put here in various bizarre costumes," that metaphor for the disabled identity is minoritizing at its core, and the internalized normate self on which it relies has a high cost for a disabled person. If he or she accepts that notion of being a "regular person" just *disguised* as disabled, the result is a failure to be recognized—either by others or even by oneself—as fundamentally human *in one's disability*.[18]

If a fundamental principle of sitting meditation is continual refusal of all categories and judgments in service of a return to an embodied, present experience, this practice cannot be complete if the embodied self is assumed to be normate. In "Unspeakable Conversations, Or How I Spent One Day as a Token Cripple at Princeton University," Harriet McBryde Johnson recounts her debate with Peter Singer over assisted suicide and euthanasia of disabled newborns. Johnson is a disability-rights activist and attorney; Singer is a philosopher whose appointment to the faculty of Princeton University stirred controversy because he advocates both animal rights and the euthanizing of disabled newborn human beings. The article juxtaposes a detailed narrative of the physical obstacles Johnson must overcome to deliver her lecture at Princeton (repairing her wheelchair when it is damaged in transit, finding an accessible hotel room, arranging for food she can swallow, navigating an inaccessible college campus, and so on) with a minutely observed response to Singer himself. She concludes with the surprised awareness that she doesn't hate Singer or find him repellent. The cost would be too great: "If I define Singer's kind of disability prejudice as an ultimate evil, and him as a monster, then I must so define all who believe disabled lives are inherently worse off . . . I can't refuse the monster-majority basic respect and human sympathy."[19]

Disability activist James Overboe challenges Johnson's refusal to condemn Singer: "As a sociologist my work centers on how humanism continues to devalue the vitalism of physical, emotional, intellectual and psychiatric disabilities in the name of a 'common sense' and normality. And Singer's position, along with other forms of humanism that promise a better world, like eugenics or the human genome project, all point to a conflation of liberal individualism (choice) and the longing for a nostalgic 'normal' community."[20] Overboe's point is that the attempt to achieve inclusion in the human community produces a repression of the phenomenological presence of disability, and at a cost: "I have been accepted by others because of my intellectual ability, but at a cost—I cannot embrace my cerebral palsy and its spasms that are a central part of me. . . . When I am caught up in the 'madness' of humanism by someone allowing me to join them I defer to them and humanism and continually find myself censoring my disabled vitality and losing my authentic voice and presence."[21]

Overboe argues, "Our experience of disability must be embraced in order for there to be the creation of a new meaning of life."[22] The phrase recalls Milam's fifth stage of the CripZen experience, the paradoxical "I am that I am," as well as Tollifson's insight on her last meditation retreat: "Somehow for me these days there's a much more profound power in allowing things not to be okay. . . . These specters that we think will be the death of us turn out to be straw tigers in the end. What we are fundamentally does not get hurt, rejected, or killed" (202–3). By the conclusion of *Bare-Bones Meditation*, Tollifson has moved beyond the notion that she has a "regular self" beneath her "bizarre costume." Instead, she embraces her most stigmatized self, asking "Is it so terrible, really, to be an ugly, depressed cripple?" (203).

There are some problematic implications for disability activism in this embrace of *what is*—"allowing things not to be okay"—associated with the meditative encounter with emptiness. While the affirmation of her most socially discredited self signals Tollifson's acceptance of disability on an individual level, she does not move to the next level, to realize that human consciousness is relational, "immanent in the living body and the interpersonal social world."[23] This realization of *interbeing*—the term used by Vietnamese Buddhist teacher Thich Nhat Hanh—gives rise to the political and ethical understanding that all human experience, including the experience of disability, incorporates, implicates, and exists in relation to both the natural environment and human society. Tollifson's use of Buddhist dharma to achieve personal peace in the face of pain is heartening. Still, how much more would she have benefited

from the teachings of engaged Buddhism, which might have shown her
a way to reclaim the activist passion that led her to disability consciousness in the first place?

Philip Martin's *The Zen Path through Depression*

Can an exploration of the temporal and spatial qualities of depression also serve as a disability narrative? We can explore this question
by considering the memoir of Philip Martin, who found himself at age
thirty-seven unexpectedly struggling with a severe depression. A psychotherapist and psychiatric social worker who had devoted "over a
decade working with people dealing with mental illness, including a
great number with depression," Martin did not initially even have a
name for what he was feeling. Nor could he find for himself the
compassion and understanding he displayed towards his clients, whom
he "encouraged . . . to keep an open mind about things such as
counseling and medication" (87). Instead, he reports, "I felt that surely
my own depression was the result of some weakness on my part, and
that I did not need any outside help" (87). Although people tried to
confront him with "what was obvious to everyone else," it was not
until his three-year-old son asked him simply "Daddy, are you not
happy?" that he finally broke through his isolation and denial (11). Only
then could Martin draw on his years of Buddhist meditation and
respond to his depression with what is called "beginner's mind": not
categorizing it or attempting to fix it, but simply experiencing it as it
was in the moment.

In *The Zen Path through Depression*, Martin recounts the experience
of becoming lost while on a canoe trip with two friends, in the
wilderness of Northern Ontario, Canada, when he was seventeen years
old. "A long rapids and waterfall were not where they were supposed
to be, and there seemed to be a lake where one shouldn't have been.
We were lost in unfamiliar territory, and our maps, and all the other
resources we depended on within ourselves, were useless" (xi). At
thirty-seven, depression plunged him in an experience of isolation,
disorientation, and inability to rely on and control his own resources
that reminded him of that camping trip. Indeed, Martin suggests that
his depression may have resulted from a survival mechanism first
developed by that teenaged self, a philosophy he had hoped "would
shield me from pain in my life. . . . I called mine the Outward Bound
approach to life. Like the people in those solo survival exercises,

outfitted only with a fishing line, a safety pin, and a match, I resolved to make it through life entirely on my own. I would depend on nothing and no one except myself" (58).

The Zen Path through Depression is a map to a territory that is both specific to one disability—the psychological and psychiatric disorder that is major depression—and also characteristic of the universal challenge articulated in the couplet from Dante that serves as Martin's epigraph: "in the middle of the path through life, / I suddenly found myself in a dark wood" (xi). While his book can be appreciated by anyone who has experienced depression, it draws specifically on the conceptual and emotional structure of Zen Buddhism. Martin studied at the Minnesota Zen Center with Dainin Katagiri Roshi, the Dharma successor to Shunryu Suzuki. *The Zen Path through Depression* consists of a series of "explorations" of the experiences of pain, impermanence, death, fear, desire, doubt, grief, the desire for escape from pain, the habit of discrimination, and anger. Martin establishes a theme for each meditation session based on one of the "Four Noble Truths," the fundamental teachings about the nature of all human experience: the existence of suffering, the origin of suffering, the cessation of suffering, and the path to the cessation of suffering.[24] Each chapter addresses the role the specific experience (of pain, of impermanence, of awareness of death, for example) plays in depression and offers a suggestion for "further exploration" that consists in merely observing the experience without judging, fighting, or attempting to control it. Modeling the encounter with depression on the encounter with no-self that is the core of meditation, Martin presents exercises through which the meditator can explore the psychic, physiological, social, and spiritual territory that depression reveals, *before* moving into any explanatory or curative response.

Perhaps because Martin is dealing not with the visible physical immobility, pain, and sexual isolation of postpolio paralysis, or the visual difference and stigma of Tollifson's missing hand, but rather the invisible mental immobility, pain, stigma, and social isolation of depression, he does not explicitly use the term "disability" to characterize his depression. Unlike Milam and Tollifson, Martin never explicitly self-identifies as disabled. Rather, he turns to the Buddhist notion of the "middle path" as a useful model for his condition: "[T]he middle path walks the line between . . . seeing existence as real and seeing it as an illusion. This middle path is a difficult path to follow, because it is utterly dynamic. It often requires us to hold two contradictory ideas in our minds at the same time. It means balancing on the razor's edge, and avoiding the temptation of easy answers" (81). As Martin applies the concept of the middle path to his depression, it produces consequences that are material, social, and medical:

> In our struggle with depression, this can mean standing in the midst of uncertainty. The uncertainty between solving all our problems with medication, and refusing to consider medication as an option. The uncertainty between viewing depression as merely a physical illness, and viewing it as a condition brought on by psychological conditions and poor coping skills. The uncertainty between working hard to heal, and just letting go and giving up trying to force a solution. (82)

How do we understand Martin's reluctance to identify as disabled? We could understand it as residue of his chosen identity as a therapist—someone who helps others rather than being helped—as well as a symptom of the shock of loss of mastery entailed by the forced surrender of such an identity. Certainly when Baba Ram Dass (Richard Alpert) had a stroke in his sixties, he felt discomfort at being forcibly evicted from the helping role, as he acknowledges in his memoir, *Still Here*. Yet the significance of that experience, Ram Dass argues, lies in exploring what the transition from helper to helped can teach one.[25] For Martin too, I would argue, his previous role as therapist coupled with his present experience of depression enables a release from recourse to labels, whether to pathologize or to normalize.

Despite their different levels of identification as disabled, however, all three writers use the experience of meditation to move from a specific focus on their impairment to a broader understanding that physical vulnerability is fundamental to all lives. As Tobin Siebers puts it: "The cycle of life runs in actuality from disability to temporary ability back to disability, and that only if you are among the most fortunate, among those who do not fall ill or suffer a severe accident. . . . It has often been claimed that the disabled body represents the image of the Other. In fact, the able body is the true image of the Other."[26] What their narratives do not seem to explore fully, however, is the means by which an encounter with one's own vulnerability and connectedness to others can provide a position from which to launch a critique of the social construction of disability as well as a program for remediating social action.

The Meditating Practitioner

What if we turn from the perspective of disabled people to the perspective of those Others—the medical and psychological personnel who *treat* the disabled, using meditation to that end? From examining how the practice of meditation reconfigures and illuminates the nature of disability as identity, I now ask how the therapeutic use of meditation shifts the conception (and experience) of identity (in particular, the response to *difference*) deployed in medical practice. I make this move, from memoir to medical treatment narrative, deliberately in order to resist the belief that experience figures as a category worth exploring only in pathographies or disability memoirs, whereas medical treatment narratives are objective and nonexperiential.

Two recent studies reporting on the use of meditation as the core of a medical treatment program for illnesses ranging from psoriasis, cancer, heart conditions, and rheumatoid arthritis to asthma and major depression demonstrate that the identity of the medical practitioner undergoes a reformulation as marked as that we found with disabled meditators. These texts, Jon Kabat-Zinn's *Full Catastrophe Living* and the less evocatively titled *Mindfulness-Based Cognitive Therapy for Depression: A New Approach to Preventing Relapse*, by Zindel V. Segal, J. Mark G. Williams, and John D. Teasdale, demonstrate a new mode of medical practice much more responsive to (and respectful of) a wide range of cultural and biological differences.[27] They also embody the beginnings of a hybrid textual genre yoking a scientific presentation of protocol for medical treatment to a more diverse aesthetic and performative narrative of individual and even collective identity transformation.

Where does difference fit into this new paradigm for health care? Difference of all kinds is understood as a crucial, and previously unacknowledged, factor in illness causation. "There are many diseases whose origins . . . are intimately linked to social factors such as poverty and social exploitation, dangerous working conditions, stressful and poisonous environmental conditions, and culturally entrenched habits, all of which are outside the direct influence of medicine and science as they are presently organized."[28] Indeed, Kabat-Zinn's book can be understood as a boundary object between the worlds of mindfulness meditation training and clinical medicine, as evidenced by the mix of professionals whose praise is quoted on the back cover: four physicians (one on the faculty of Harvard Medical School), the director of an addictive behavior research center, and the founding head of the Insight Meditation Society (Barre, Massachusetts).[29] A new openness to difference extends to discursive conventions, too. Both the texts of Kabat-Zinn and Segal et al. combine the reevaluation of categories with what I have called discursive hybridity. By this I do *not* mean that they co-opt Eastern spirituality into the Western medical paradigm, although that is arguable, but rather that they incorporate aspects of traditionally literary and humanistic discourses into the framework of medical science. So Kabat-Zinn's book transcends the cultural and disciplinary boundaries that have allocated medicine to the realm of positivist instrumentality while confining literature to the realm of aesthetic value enhancement, from its title *Full Catastrophe Living*, drawn from *Zorba the Greek*, to its concluding citation of Pablo Neruda's poem "Keeping Quiet." Moreover, the generic hybridity is intimately related to the reversal of perspective that the book advocates. Just as the disability narratives discussed earlier portray how the experience of disability has—through the practice of meditation—opened out to an understanding of the impermanence, vulnerability, and dependency central to all lives, so here the use of meditation as a medical treatment opens out from the narrow focus on illness, pain, and loss of control to a broader project of integrating the vicissitudes inevitable in life within an experience of health and well-being.

Similarly, *Mindfulness-Based Cognitive Therapy for Depression* by Segal, Williams, and Teasdale reveals both medical and discursive innovation. The three cognitive psychologists who wrote the study made the specific decision to depart from the standard scientific publication format. Instead they recount the following:

> The story of their own learning in encountering and then testing a very different paradigm from that in which they were trained professionally and in which they were recognized as experts. This is an unusual approach for a scientific text, as the authors themselves acknowledge, and one that . . . is, in this instance, both admirable and totally appropriate to accomplish their professional purposes given the subject matter.[30]

This work echoes the generic hybridity of *Full Catastrophe Living*, being both commercially and formally innovative. In addition to including the charts, tables, and handouts accompanying the eight sessions of therapeutic exercises used in the clinical trial, it even grants the purchaser a "Limited Photocopy License," specifying that those pages, tables, and charts may be reproduced by "qualified mental health professionals" for use with their own clients and patients (copyright page). Then, in a move beyond the disciplinary exclusivity of that limited license, the authors introduce poems, autobiographical narratives, Middle-Eastern teaching stories, and what might be called a scientific parable, as well as an extremely accessible popular-science explanation of "the power of randomization" and the procedure they followed in their randomized clinical trial, to broaden its address beyond clinicians to a general audience.

As a result of those scaled innovations, what begins as a distinctly minoritizing construction of disability develops into a universalizing one. Or, to put it another way, what began as a text addressed to physicians and psychologists for treating patients and clients becomes a text addressing anyone who has experienced a life reorientation leading to a broader sense of self. Beginning with the desire to help their clients, previously disabled by depression, from experiencing a relapse, the three psychologists explain how they became motivated to change their own professional and personal practices, not only applying a meditation model drawn from Eastern religion to their Western medical practices, but taking up mindfulness meditation themselves. Though we are now in the realm of clinical case study rather than pathography or disability narrative, once again we find the focus on mindfulness catalyzes the transcendence of specific identity categories. As Segal et al. observe, "A commonality of experience crosses the usual boundaries between researchers, clinicians, and patients. Each has made discoveries from which he or she learned. . . . As it turns out, the wisdom that helps us to deal with tragedies and disappointments is the same wisdom that sees, in the ordinary and everyday things of life, how things change from one moment to the next, often in surprising ways."[31]

The insight that meditation enables is thus inherently political. Not only does meditation challenge what Lennard Davis has character-ized as "the fantasy of culture, democracy, capitalism, sexism, and racism, to name only a few ideologies, [that one can attain] the perfection of the body and its activities," but when linked to a socially engaged Buddhism it can also support work to eradicate the social and political oppression bred by such ideologies.[32] Of course, as we move from the inevitably limited individual body to those large institutions aspiring to its improvement (and fantasizing its perfection), just as we ask questions about the context in which impairment becomes disability, so too we must ask questions about the context in which meditation becomes medicine. Eve Kosofsky Sedgwick has eloquently traced the paradox inherent in the affective embrace of Buddhist thinking:

The Western reader drawn to Buddhist pedagogical thinking may be most at risk of decontextualizing and misrecognizing it, riding roughshod over its cultural difference, even recasting it in her own image—the worst Orientalizing vices identified by recent critical scholarship—just to the degree that she can apprehend it through a Buddhist sense of knowing rather than a Western one. Conversely, from within the framework of the Buddhist respect for realization as both dense process and active practice, a theorized scholarly skepticism as to whether Buddhism can be known by Westerners may reveal its own dependence on an eerily thin Western phenomenology of "knowing."[33]

Thus a westerner who feels drawn to Buddhism may be deeply realizing Buddhist dharma precisely by seeing it "as not other than oneself," even when such an act of recognition seems like the most blatant sort of cultural appropriation. Following that insight, I am more interested now in the instrumental, scientific deployment of meditation in medicine than in making the obvious point about its cultural decontextualization.

As Davis's reference to broader institutional and ideological forces indicates, we stop short if we focus only on meditation's effect on individuals, whether the disabled individual seeking relief from her/his disability, or the able physician or psychologist seeking to provide that relief. There will be limitations to the identity transformations enabled by Zen meditation precisely because of its position within a sociocultural and economic field. The multiplication of for-profit alternative medicine centers testifies to the fact that meditation, like medication, is increasingly commodified. Because the work of Segal et al. is informed by a public health perspective, its use of meditation must be considered in that context. Meditation is targeted to a specific population: people who have suffered at least one episode of major depression (or as many as three) and who are at risk of a relapse. The authors comment explicitly on the cost- and time-effective nature of group instruction in meditation, yoga, and other body-based mindfulness technique methods, which can treat a large number of people for the cost and time that would otherwise be used for one person in individual psychotherapy. They offer little space for the explicitly individually oriented perspectives familiar from the narratives by Milam, Tollifson, and Martin. Nor do they adopt a broader systemwide perspective that might be critical of a society that relies on mindfulness training to repair the damages wrought by demanding, high-intensity careers focused on personal or collective productivity rather than personal or collective meaning.[34]

Similarly, Philip Martin's exploration of the efficacy of meditation is shaped and constrained by the broader institutional structures of disciplinary and professional identity and commodification. Martin's brave assertion of a liminal identity as a person with depression *and* as a therapist is enabled by his encounter with Zen meditation only to be undercut by the publisher's defensive marketing department, which emphasizes Martin's professional status in its choice of book design. While the text of Martin's book maps the middle path between a minoritizing and a universalizing view of depression, the publication format ultimately closes off that productive liminal zone with a prefatory disclaimer firmly resituating Martin in the position of health-care provider, subjecting his reader to the regulatory discourses of medicine and law: "While the techniques described in this book may alleviate symptoms of depression in some individuals, depression is a serious illness that may in some cases require medical treatment by a licensed health-care professional, and readers are encouraged to seek such advice. Neither the author nor the publisher assumes any liability for any injury that may be suffered by any person applying the techniques set forth in this book" (vi).

The impairment/disability system "the process by which biological impairment is transformed into cultural disability"—plays out very differently in Martin's narrative than it does in Tollifson's gradual encounter with the psychic and social meaning of her missing hand and Milam's furiously funny acknowledgement of his battle with his own self-pity and the condescension of others.[35] The crucial difference between them is the degree to which they are willing to identify as disabled. Ironically, it is precisely Martin's professional ability as a psychotherapist that may make him unwilling to claim identity as disabled, or to take refuge in the privilege of the physician. The normalizing model still available (in fantasy) to those like Milam and Tollifson who suffer from bodily impairment is not accessible to those who, like Martin, suffer from mental impairment. The prefatory proviso with its careful attention to the potential medical and legal implications of Martin's advice is "symptomatic of a larger, cultural anxiety surrounding mental illness" that produces materially different identity positions for the mentally and the physically disabled.[36] This is not to argue that mental and physical disabilities are so easily disentangled, of course. All too often people with physical disabilities are treated as though they are cognitively or psychologically impaired as well. Yet to the extent that we can tease them apart, it is worth considering the different social stigma attached—particularly in a clinical or therapeutic

setting—to mental disability. Not only does the discourse of the democratic citizen privilege the intact and autonomous self, but the discourse
of medicine figures mental illness as an irreparable, symbolically freighted
breach in self-determination. In order for Martin's book to be of use to
the reader desiring clinical guidance, it must be written by someone in
command of his faculties.

Disability Koans

This brings me back to the questions with which I began: What
experience of identity does meditation catalyze, and what are the
implications for disability studies? As I mentioned at the outset, I
practice meditation. I began meditating over five years ago, as a way
of traversing territory similar to the wilderness that Philip Martin
mapped in *The Zen Path through Depression*. In my case the depression
followed a painful illness and surgery; through it I have come to know
well the genetic and psychic pathways that Martin charts. Do I identify
as disabled? That identity oscillates for me, mirroring my changing
meditation spaces: in Pennsylvania, a corner in my study; in New York
City, a closet in a small apartment. At times, I certainly have so
identified: when I have been unable to think clearly because of depression, when my ability to work has vanished into the sludge of fatigue
and uncertainty, or when my passion for adventure and play has fizzled
out in a drab calm. But at other times, that label has seemed not only
incomplete but actually unhelpful because it truncates the sense of
spacious possibility that I experience in meditation. And in those times,
with Lorenzo Milam, I resist any label at all, preferring perhaps "I am
that I am," even as I laugh or wince at the echo of the Old Testament
in the phrase.

Moreover, the indeterminate or variable construction of identity
links my experience to the texts I have been considering. Though
Tollifson, Milam, and Martin may have turned to meditation as a relief
from the pain of their disability, and though Kabat-Zinn and Segal et
al. may have deployed meditation as a form of medical treatment, what
each group found was less a confirmation of the identity position with
which they began (as disabled individuals or as medical practitioners)
than a dissolution of that identity, an understanding of its inherent
impermanence. To put it another way, the lesson I learned through
illness, surgery, and depression was the same one that both the disabled
meditators and the meditation-based medical practitioners learned, and

articulated, in the course of their narratives. Lennard Davis expresses the insight as follows: "What is universal in life, if there are universals, is the experience of the limitations of the body."[37] Because of my experiences with meditation, I note and surrender the identity of disability, understanding it as both characterizing and escaping the moment-to-moment experience of being myself.

What does that oscillating affiliation with disability identity signify, in social and intellectual terms? I would venture first that it marks a high-stakes conflict in disability studies between a rejection of the normate when it is framed as morphological and a privileging of the normate when it is framed as psychological. To put the issue bluntly, if a scholar claims mental disability, and identifies as mentally disabled, can he or she still work as effectively in disability studies? As a scholar? As an activist? Will the university and publishing apparatus within which her/his claims must be made value them commensurately to those of a mentally able, or at least effectively closeted, individual? As one scholar with Tourette's syndrome said to me, "If I came out as having Tourette's, the legitimacy of all of my work would be called into question." What price disability identity, when the disability is psychological, in a profession that so highly values intellectual clarity and rationality?[38]

However, what of Kay Redfield Jamison, the clinical psychologist who has written so bravely and insightfully about her own bipolar disorder?[39] One reader of this essay suggested that Jamison's successful career proves that such a dual identification—as mentally disabled person and as professional practitioner/scholar—is viable. In contrast, I would argue that Jamison's iconic status as what some call a "Supercrip" (that is, someone who *although disabled* performs better than a nondisabled, "normal" person) is the exception that proves the rule. Her fame testifies to the difficulty of drawing on one's professional authority in service of a devalued and discredited social position.[40] Moreover, physician Steven Miles's experience of investigation by his professional licensing board following his disclosure that he suffered from "type II bipolar disorder, a mainly depressive disorder, unaccompanied by life-disrupting mania" reveals that nonpsychiatrist medical practitioners are similarly jeopardized.[41]

Yet if it is professionally risky to come out as a psychologically or cognitively disabled person, there are dangers lurking in the closet as well. If a disability studies scholar remains closeted as someone who has experienced mental illness (be it depression, schizophrenia, obsessive compulsive disorder, bipolar disorder), how authoritative or legitimate can that disabilities scholarship be? What are the gains and losses in that act of closeting for those in the disability studies community? What is the ethical and political significance of that choice?

Perhaps we shouldn't dismiss the example of Kay Jamison. What if we think of it not as enabling an affirmation of disability identification, but as unsettling the stark binary nature of any identity at all? To frame the choice for those who experience psychological disability as a simple binary one—stay closeted as a person with a disability or "come out" as mentally disabled—may be to miss the point. If we expand the disability studies paradigm to reincorporate the insights that Zen meditation has made possible, we can ask ourselves what the implications are of categorizing ourselves in terms of any aspect of mind-body experience.

What do we lose when we refuse our encounter with the imperfect, disabled, physically and/or mentally limited aspects of our embodied selves—those aspects that are *inevitably* part of living as temporal beings? What "important political and ethical work" do we dodge when we refuse that encounter? Conversely, when we use those aspects to define ourselves, how have we silenced our experiences as selves that are strong, able, and richly alive? What is the personal, even spiritual price of that tactically important political and ethical act? What moments of meaning, what encounters with wisdom do we thus forgo when we accept the stasis of a label? Conversely, what are the effects of that refusal on our scholarship, *whatever our identification*? How might that refusal be of a piece with the motive to normalize and pathologize, or to cling to the fantasy of a perfect self by positing a rejected, physically and/or mentally imperfect Other? These are not so much questions to answer, or even problems to solve, than they are *koans*: intellectual, social, legal, and ethical paradoxes, arising from the experience of disability, that merit our collective meditation.

NOTES

My thanks to Jonathan Metzl and Suzanne Poirier, to the readers for *Literature and Medicine*, and to the Six Rings Sangha.
    1. According to Zen Master Dogen, when one learns the "essential art of zazen" then the "body-mind of itself will drop off and your original face will appear." Zen Master Dogen, "Recommending Zazen to All People," in *Enlightenment Unfolds: The Essential Teachings of Zen Master Dogen*, ed. Kazuaki Tanahashi (Boston: Shambhala, 2000), 32–3. In her discussion of the issue of surgical modification of the faces of children with Down's syndrome, Janet Lyon has identified another site where a conversation between Buddhism and disability would be illuminating. There is important tension between the Zen model of seeing one's original face and the "long historical effort on the part of normative culture to avoid ethical contact with the face of disability, with the face of the other . . . with the face of 'irrevocable difference.'"

Janet Lyon, "About Faces and Down Syndrome," paper, "Ethics and Disability Lecture Series," Rock Ethics Institute, Penn State University, University Park, PA, March 24, 2003.

2. Lorenzo Wilson Milam, *CripZen: A Manual for Survival* (San Diego, CA: MHO and MHO WORKS, 1993). Subsequent references are cited parenthetically in the text.

3. Joan Tollifson, *Bare-Bones Meditation: Waking Up from the Story of My Life* (New York: Bell Tower, 1992). Subsequent references are cited parenthetically in the text.

4. Philip Martin, *The Zen Path through Depression* (San Francisco: HarperSanFrancisco, 1999). Subsequent references are cited parenthetically in the text.

5. Jon Kabat-Zinn, *Full Catastrophe Living* (New York: Delta, 1990); and Zindel V. Segal, J. Mark G. Williams, and John D. Teasdale, *Mindfulness-Based Cognitive Therapy for Depression: A New Approach to Preventing Relapse* (New York: Guildford Press, 2002).

6. An issue that requires an essay to itself is the role meditation plays in negotiating the identities of disability and race. One might compare to these three narratives by white disabled meditators a recent surge in meditation narratives by African American authors, most notably Alice Walker and bell hooks. Walker began studying TM (Transcendental Meditation) when she was living in New York City after a divorce. She went on to study *tonglen* (the Tibetan Buddhist practice of meditation) with teacher Pema Chodron, with whom she has engaged in many public dialogues, including the audiotape *Pema Chodron and Alice Walker in Conversation: On the Meaning of Suffering and the Mystery of Joy.* hooks, whose *All About Love: New Visions* came out in 2000 and *Salvation: Black People and Love* in 2002, has been a practicing Buddhist since she was an eighteen-year-old Stanford undergraduate. In a recent interview with *Tricycle: The Buddhist Review,* hooks articulated a concept of identity with remarkable resonances to the argument I am making here: "If I were really asked to define myself, I wouldn't start with race; I wouldn't start with blackness; I wouldn't start with gender; I wouldn't start with feminism. I would start with stripping down to what fundamentally informs my life, which is that I'm a seeker on the path. I think of feminism, and I think of anti-racist struggles as part of it. But where I stand spiritually is, steadfastly, on a path about love." Helen Tworkov, "Agents of Change: An Interview with bell hooks," *Tricycle: The Buddhist Review* 2, no. 1 (1992): 48–57. For the disabled meditators I discuss in this essay, as for hooks, this is a love that extends not only to others but to the self in its embodied and experienced specificity.

7. Lennard Davis, *Bending Over Backwards: Disability, Dismodernism, and Other Difficult Positions* (New York: New York University Press, 2002), 1.

8. Eva Kittay, "Caring for the Vulnerable by Caring for the Caregiver: The Case of Mental Retardation," (paper, Rock Ethics Institute, Penn State, University Park, PA, March 15, 2002).

9. James I. Charlton, *Nothing About Us Without Us: Disability Oppression and Empowerment* (Berkeley: University of California Press, 1998), 4.

10. As Wendy Brown's work would suggest, precisely the attempt to redress marginalization reinstantiates the process producing it, in the act of making the claim. Wendy Brown, *States of Injury: Power and Freedom in Late Modernity* (Princeton: Princeton University Press, 1995), 7.

11. Donna J. Haraway, *Simians, Cyborgs, and Women: The Reinvention of Nature* (New York: Routledge, 1991), 111.

12. Lorenzo Wilson Milam, *The Cripple Liberation Front Marching Band Blues* (San Diego CA: MHO and MHO WORKS, 1984).

13. Milam references Appendix II, where he glosses this phrase, which in the Book of Exodus is the name of God. "I-am-that-I-am. A statement directly out of Buddhism: paradoxical, saying everything and nothing, leaving us to contemplate the

glorious contradictions that are as much the problem of our lives as our unstable reliance on words" (223).

14. The full passage is comically paradoxical:

"I really don't care what they give me for a body, as long as they don't make me come back as me any more," I said. "You know I like myself well enough, have had fairly good times with me (some bad times, too). . . .

"'I've done with that one,' I'll tell them. 'You want me to be divine don't you? Well, give me something nice to be divine in for a change.'" . . . .

"I'll be good, I promise you," I'll tell them. "I'll give up everything when I get through with the usual teen-age indiscretions. After just a few short years, I'll become a holy man, a wandering saddhu. I promise faithfully: I'll spend the rest of my years cheerfully walking the land, delivering Lordly messages, eating bark and drinking nothing stronger than leaf tea and branchwater, pausing only briefly near the beaches to look . . . at the figure I once was, the one I once wanted to be.

"I am sure that after they hear my plea," I tell her, "they'll be more than willing to trust me with a new, powerful, lithe body—so I can have some fun for the first few years of my new return, before I turn into the saint they (and all of us) can be so proud of." (250–1)

15. Her California friend's joke about her German shepherd as "the one in the dog suit" suggests the potentially profound reframing of identity that meditation enables, challenging not just the categories for human beings (race, age, sex, ability) but the category of species as well.

16. Rosemarie Garland-Thomson, *Extraordinary Bodies: Figuring Physical Disability in American Culture and Literature* (New York: Columbia University Press, 1997), 8.

17. Ibid.

18. Paradoxical indeed that we would actually *prefer* to maintain our human privilege by disavowing aspects of human behavior that are not rational or under our control than to extend our sense of fellow feeling to members of other species.

19. Harriet McBryde Johnson, "Unspeakable Conversations, Or How I Spent One Day as a Token Cripple at Princeton University," *New York Times Magazine*, February 16, 2003, Section 6: 50–5, 74, 78–9, 79.

20. James Overboe, posting on the DS-HUM listserv, 12:30 pm, February 16, 2003, http://listserv.umd.edu/cgi-bin/wa?A2=ind0302&L=ds-hum&P=R2496 (accessed March 18, 2004).

21. Ibid.

22. James Overboe, "'Difference in Itself': Validating Disabled People's Lived Experience," *Body and Society* 5, no. 4 (1999): 17–29, 27.

23. Evan Thompson, "Human Consciousness: From Intersubjectivity to Interbeing," http://www.philosophy.ucf.edu/pcsfetz1.html (accessed March 18, 2004). See also Thich Nhat Hahn, *Interbeing: Fourteen Guidelines for Engaged Buddhism* (Berkeley, CA.: Parallax Press, 1987).

24. Sharon Salzberg and Joseph Goldstein, *Insight Meditation* (Boulder, CO: Sounds True, 2001), 131. I agree with Eve Kosofsky Sedgwick in preferring Stephen Batchelor's reformulation of these as "active and performatively differentiated *injunctions* (to '*understanding* anguish, *letting go* of its origins, *realizing* its cessation, and *cultivating* the path')." Sedgwick, "Pedagogy of Buddhism," in *Touching Feeling: Affect, Pedagogy, Performativity* (Durham, NC: Duke University Press, 2003), 170 (Sedgwick's italics).

25. Ram Dass, *Still Here: Embracing Aging, Changing and Dying*, ed. Mark Matousek and Marlene Roeder, (New York: Riverhead Books, 2000).

26. Tobin Siebers, "Disability in Theory: From Social Constructionism to the New Realism of the Body," *American Literary History* 13, no. 4 (2001): 737–54, 742.

27. Several months after I finished this paper, the *New York Times Magazine* published Stephen S. Hall's article on neuropsychological collaborations with the Dalai Lama and other Buddhist meditators to improve immunological as well as psychological health. Hall, "Is Buddhism Good for Your Health?" *New York Times Magazine*, September 14, 2003, 46–9, http://www.nytimes.com/2003/09/14/magazine/14BUDDHISM.html (accessed on September 18, 2003).

28. Kabat-Zinn, 186.

29. I am borrowing the term "boundary object" from Geoffrey C. Bowker and Susan Leigh Starr, who use it to refer to "objects that both inhabit several communities of practice and satisfy the informational requirements of each of them . . . [are] plastic enough to adapt to local needs . . . yet robust enough to maintain a common identity across sites." *Sorting Things Out: Classification and Its Consequences* (Cambridge: MIT Press, 1999), 297. Of course, attention to cultural differences has also provided a rich reservoir of alternative healthcare practices. See Lynn Payer, *Medicine and Culture* (New York: Henry Holt, 1988). Moreover, while so-called "New Age" approaches to medicine can at times be reductive, culturally sensitive approaches to medicine can affirm the complex identities and practices of non-Western medical traditions. For a discussion of the need for such new approaches to medical care, see Anne Fadiman, *The Spirit Catches You and You Fall Down: A Hmong Child, Her American Doctors, and the Collision of Two Cultures* (New York: Farrar, Straus and Giroux: 1997), and for a discussion of the reductionism of a specific New Age treatment, see Jackie Stacey, *Teratologies: A Cultural Study of Cancer* (London: Routledge, 1997).

30. Jon Kabat-Zinn, foreword to *Mindfulness-Based Cognitive Therapy for Depression: A New Approach to Preventing Relapse*, by Segal et al., vii.

31. Ibid., 329, 332.

32. Davis, 32. For an example of how socially engaged Buddhism can take on the intersecting experiences of disability and the history of oppression based on race and gender, see Michelle T. Clinton, "Breathing Through History: A Dark Reflection on Zen," *Turning Wheel: The Journal of Socially Engaged Buddhism*, Summer 2003: 34–6.

33. Sedgwick, 168.

34. For the most powerful recent intervention in this area, see the "Take Back Your Time" movement, a project of the Center for Religion, Ethics and Social Policy at Cornell University, http://www.simpleliving.net/timeday (accessed on December 5, 2003).

35. Elizabeth J. Donaldson, "The Corpus of the Madwoman: Toward a Feminist Disability Studies Theory of Embodiment and Mental Illness," *NWSA Journal* 14, no. 3 (2002): 99–119, 111.

36. Ibid., 113.

37. Davis, 32.

38. In focusing on psychological disability I am not addressing the related, but distinctly different, issues posed by cognitive disablement. See Kate Lindemann, "Persons with Adult-Onset Head Injury: A Crucial Resource for Feminist Philosophers," *Hypatia* 16, no. 4 (Fall 2001): 105–23. I also do not consider the difficulty of being closeted with a mental disability, whether it is depression, bipolar disorder, or schizophrenia. Although morphologically invisible impairments, such illnesses produce significant—and thus often *socially perceptible*—distortions of one's ability to function well in community. However, that is for another essay.

39. Kay Redfield Jamison, *An Unquiet Mind* (New York: Alfred A. Knopf, 1995).

40. Beth Haller, "False Positive," *Ragged Edge Magazine Online*, January/February 2000, http://www.towson.edu/~bhalle/rag-article.html (accessed on September 18, 2003).

41. Steven H. Miles, "A Challenge to Licensing Boards: The Stigma of Mental Illness," *JAMA* 280, no. 10 (1998): 865.

Fat as Disability:
The Case of the Jews

Sander L. Gilman

How slippery the concept of obesity truly is can be judged, perhaps, from the following thought experiment.[1] Let us look at the question of what constitutes a "disability." Obesity is now considered a disability though for a long period of time it was not. It was only in 1993 that the federal Equal Employment Opportunity Commission ruled that "severely obese" people could claim protection under federal statutes barring discrimination against the disabled. A "friend of the court" brief based on this ruling was filed in the case of *Cook v. Rhode Island*, a suit brought by a Rhode Island woman, Bonnie Cook, who accused the state of illegally denying her a job on the basis of "perceived disability" because of her size.

The Americans with Disabilities Act (1990) states that impairment is a condition that substantially limits major life activities. (Analogous definitions are used in the Canadian Charter of Rights and Freedoms [1982], the British Disability Discrimination Act [1995], and the Swedish Act concerning Support and Services for Persons with Certain Functional Impairments [1993].) Obesity certainly does limit such activities. The obese "continually encounter various forms of discrimination, including outright intentional exclusion, the discriminatory effects of architectural, transportation, and communication barriers, overprotective rules and policies, failure to make modifications to existing facilities and practices, exclusionary qualification standards and criteria, segregation, and relegation to lesser services, programs, activities, benefits, jobs, or other opportunities."[2] Under the regulations promulgated to enforce this act, severe obesity is defined as body weight more than 100 percent over the norm and is deemed "clearly an impairment."[3] This rather arbitrary line means that to be covered by the Americans with Disabilities Act the individual cannot just be too overweight for a specific occupation but has to be morbidly obese. In one case the court held that the male "plaintiff cannot demonstrate that he was regarded as disabled on the basis of a specific job of his choosing."[4] Thus, the question of defining obesity as a disability remains fluid.

The definition of a disability seems to be rather specific even if the Supreme Court has been recently altering and limiting it. The World Health Organization (WHO), in its 1980 *International Classification of Impairments, Disabilities, and Handicaps*, makes a seemingly clear distinction among impairment, disability, and handicap. "Impairment" is an abnormality of structure or function at the organ level while "disability" is the functional consequence of such impairment. A "handicap" is the social consequence of impairment and its resultant disability. Thus, cognitive or hearing impairments may lead to communication problems, which in turn result in isolation or dependency. Such a functional approach (and this approach was long the norm in American common and legal usage) seems to be beyond any ideological bias. This changes very little in the most recent shift to the idea that disability be redefined on a scale of "human variation" that postulates the difficulties of the disabled as the result of the inflexibility of social institutions rather than their own impairment.

When, however, we substitute "obesity" for "cognitive impairment" in the functional model, there is suddenly an evident and real set of implied ethical differences in thinking about what a disability can be. What is obesity? While there are sets of contemporary medical definitions of obesity, it is also clear that these definitions change from culture to culture as well as over time. Obesity is determined by more than the body-mass index (wt/ht^2), because even this changes meaning over time.[5] Today in the United States and the United Kingdom, people with a BMI between 25–30 kg/m^2 are categorized as overweight, and those with a BMI above 30 kg/m^2 are labeled as obese. Yet the BMI that categorizes people as obese was altered in 1995 and had previously been lower.[6] What is considered fat and what obese shift over time.

Let us apply the rather straightforward WHO standards of disability to the world of the obese. Is obesity the end product of impairment or is it impairment itself? If it is impairment, what organ is "impaired"? Is it the body itself? The digestive system? The circulatory system? Or is it the mind and therefore the obese suffer from that most stigmatizing of illnesses, mental illness? Is obesity a mental illness that is the result of an addictive personality?[7] Is addiction a sign of the lack of will? Is it physical dependency, as in heroin addiction? Is addiction a genetically preprogrammed "error" in the human body, which expresses itself in psychological desire for food or the inability to recognize when one is no longer hungry?

Is the impairment of obesity like lung cancer in that it is the result of the voluntary consumption of a dangerous substance such as fat or carbohydrates? Certainly the WHO believes this. Having struggled against tobacco consumption, it is intent on launching a campaign against the rising levels of obesity by persuading manufacturers of processed foods to limit the amounts of added sugar.[8] Is such food "addictive" like nicotine, or is it merely an interchangeable sign in society for those things we all desire but most of us can limit? Surely it is not possible to go without food as one could go without cigarettes. Is the obese person mentally or physically disabled? On the other hand, can you be obese and mentally stable? Is obesity a disease of "civilization" caused by too fat or too rich or too well-processed food? Is its "cure" a return to "real" food or the rejection of food in general? Has it become the new "epidemic" to be chartered by epidemiologists and combated by public health organizations?[9] If it is an epidemic, does it reflect a single cause (such as SARS) or is it merely ubiquitous? Or is it a disease at all? As one journalist comments, "[B]eing too fat is not usually regarded as a real 'disease' by most people—even those who are."[10] What are the social consequences of obesity—isolation or a central place in society? Where on the scale of "human variation" are you placed in a world completely shaped by and for those who are not fat? Is obesity exogenous or endogenous? Are you in the end treated like a social pariah or Santa Claus?

Many years ago, H. Tristram Engelhardt, Jr., a leading medical ethicist, noted that "deciding what counts as health requires a decision about what counts as an appropriate goal for man. And to be sound, such a decision requires clear logic, breadth of reasoning, and creative sensitivity with respect to ethical issues. These are philosophical problems as much as they are medical problems."[11] I would add that these are cultural and historical problems as well and that obesity can serve as an elegant object of study for the complexities of defining the "healthy" and the "ill." The study of obesity in its cultural and social contexts provides a wide range of interlocking questions about the cultural construction of the body. The role that race plays is one further variable in the study of the cultural representation of the obese body.

Jews and Fat

Historically, the Jews placed relatively little focus on the representation of the fat body. Such a body is evoked by the biblical figure of Eglon, King of Moab, who oppressed the children of Israel for eighteen years.[12] (As the Jewish body was defined by circumcision, it was usually represented by the male body.) Judges 3:17–22 relates how his fat, male (*ish bari me' od*) body was destroyed by the left-handed hero Ehud.[13] He smuggles his sword into the presence of the king by wearing it on the "wrong-side," at least the wrong side for right-handers. Ehud is "treacherous and sneaky; perhaps the culture of ancient Israel thought those descriptions to be synonymous, or at least stereotypical."[14] As for the fat king, the text describes how Eglon's fat closed about the blade when he was pierced. His guards do not even notice that he has been disemboweled until they smell his feces. Is this the case of one deviant body destroying another? The Talmudic fat male body is a deviant one, but not particularly a dangerous one. Rather, it holds a certain fascination.

The idea that the fat body thinks intuitively is an inherent aspect of Talmudic discourse. Indeed, in one of the books of the Talmud, *Baba Metzia* 83b–85a, so ably explicated by Daniel Boyarin, the tale of Rabbi El'azar, the son of Shim'on, reveals that El'azar intuitively knows the truth because of his fat body. As a Roman "quisling," he makes judgments that seem destructive, arbitrary, or foolish, but because he knows the truth intuitively, he is always right. He is a fat sleuth, whose solutions turn out always to be accurate even though at first glance they appear to be false. One day, he has a "certain laundry man," who had insulted him, arrested. Before he can come to his senses, the man is hanged. As Rabbi El'azar stands below the body and weeps for his error, he is told that the man had violated a number of *mitzvoth* (laws) that would have condemned him to death anyway. When his judgment is so affirmed, "he placed his hands on his guts and said: 'Be joyful, O my guts, be joyful! If it is thus when you are doubtful, when you are certain even more so. I am confident that rot and worms cannot prevail over you.'" But in spite of this, he remains unconvinced of his inherent, fat facility. When he is drugged, "baskets of fat" are ripped from his gut and placed in the July sun. "And it did not stink. But no fat stinks. It does if it has red blood vessels in it, and this even though it had red blood vessels in it, did not stink."[15] It is the belly, now separate from the body, which has a life of its own. It represents the intuitive ability of this otherwise suspect figure to judge truth from falsity; it is a gut feeling, quite literally.

Jewish attitudes toward obesity were clearly defined by the model of the lack of self-control. Unlike its inclusion in the much later Christian theology's enumeration of the "Seven Deadly Sins," gluttony is not included in either version of the Ten Commandments presented in the Hebrew bible. Gluttony is, of course, not praised among the Jews. It can be seen as a sign of human failing, as in Proverbs 23:20–1 ("Be not among winebibbers; among riotous eaters of flesh; For the drunkard and the glutton shall come to poverty: and drowsiness shall clothe a man with rags"), or of disobedience to God, as in Deuteronomy 21:20 ("This our son is stubborn and rebellious, he will not obey our voice; he is a glutton, and a drunkard; And all the men of his city shall stone him with stones, that he die").[16] It is only with the Pauline condemnation of the flesh that the desecration of the "temple of the Holy Ghost" through obesity stains the soul that inhabits the obese body. The fat man is unable to become truly righteous. (I Corinthians 6:19: "What? know ye not that your body is the temple of the Holy Ghost which is in you, which ye have of God, and ye are not your own?")

Obesity among the Jews living in the Christian and Moslem Diaspora was a sign of the lack of self-discipline inappropriate for a real man, a real scholar, and it could be punished.[17] In the classic work of the twelfth-century Iberian physician-philosopher Maimonides on dietetics, the *Regimen of Health*, there is no sense that obesity was a moral or even a medical problem (at least for the rulers for whom he wrote) whereas he does note sexual overexertion as one.[18] However, obesity was still viewed as an important health issue with repercussions upon the body of the individual; Maimonides treated the condition of "obese old men" with medication, exercise, massage, and baths.[19] His work provides a synthesis of Galenic medicine and the work of the Arabic physician Ibn Sina (known in the West as Avicenna, 980–1037), whose *Kitah al-Quanun*, or *The Canon*, includes a detailed discussion of obesity in its fourth book.

It is only in modernity that the Jew's body comes to represent all of the potential for disease and decay associated with the modern body of the fat male. In modern medicine, there has been a preoccupation with a claimed Jewish predisposition to diabetes. The nineteenth-century practice of labeling Jews as a "diabetic" race was a means of labeling them as inferior. In the fall of 1888, the Parisian neurologist Jean-Martin Charcot described to Sigmund Freud the predisposition of Jews for specific forms of illness, such as diabetes, and how "the exploration is easy" because the illness was caused by consanguineous marriage among the Jews. Jewish "incest" left its mark on the Jewish body, as well as on the Jewish soul, in the form of diabetes. (Indicative of his deprecatory attitude in regard to the Jews, Charcot's letter to Freud used the vulgar *juif* rather than the more polite *Israélite* or more scientific *sémite*.[20]) However, there are further views on why the Jews are predisposed to this illness. The British eugenicist George Pitt-Rivers attributed the increased rate of diabetes among the Jews to "the passionate nature of their temperaments." He noted that by the 1920s diabetes was commonly called a "Jewish disease."[21]

Over and over again it was the obesity inherent in the Jew's body (and soul) that was seen as the cause of the illness. The "Oriental races, enervated by climate, customs, and a super-alimentation abounding in fats, sugar and pastry will inevitably progress towards the realization of fat generations, creating an extremely favourable soil for obesity."[22] Even in the Diaspora, the assumption is that the Jew is diabetic because of his predisposition for fat: "All observers are agreed that Jews are specially liable to become diabetic. . . . A person belonging to the richer classes in towns usually eats too much, spends a great part of his life indoors; takes too little bodily exercise, and overtakes his nervous system in the pursuit of knowledge, business, or pleasure. . . . Such a description is a perfectly accurate account of the well-to-do Jew, who raises himself easily by his superior mental ability to a comfortable social position, and notoriously avoids all kinds of bodily exercise."[23] Jews inherited their tendency toward fat because of their lifestyle: "Can a surfeit of food continued through many generations create large appetites in the offspring; alternatively, can it cause a functional weakness of their weight-regulating mechanism?" asks William F. Christie. And he answers:

Take, for instance, the Hebrews, scattered over the ends of the earth. Probably no race in the world has so apparent a tendency to become stout after the age of puberty, or is more frequently cited as an example of racial adiposity. It is also probable that no nation is so linked in common serfdom to their racial habits and customs. [Elliot] Joslin says of the present generation of Jews: "Overeating begins in childhood, and lasts till old age." The inheritance of large appetites and depressed weight-regulating mechanism may exist in them, although they show no other signs of the latter; whereas the inheritance of fat-forming habits is certain.[24]

Here "nature" trumps "culture" even among emancipated Jews.

Thus, Jews inherit the compulsive eating patterns of their ancestors and are therefore fat already as children. Their obesity and their diabetes are a reflection of their poor hygienic traditions, precisely the opposite of the claims of nineteenth-century Jewish reformers who saw Judaism as the rational religion of hygiene. Indeed, it is the "Oriental"

Jew who presents the worst-case scenario for this line of argument. Max Oertel, perhaps the most quoted authority on obesity at the beginning of the twentieth century, states that "[t]he Jewesses of Tunis when barely ten years old are systematically fattened by being confined in dark narrow rooms and fed with farinaceous articles and the flesh of young dogs, until in the course of a few months they resemble shapeless lumps of fat."[25] Here the Western fantasy about the "Oriental" body is heightened by the Jews feeding their daughters nonkosher food. Jews, according to much of the late nineteenth-century literature critical of Jewish ritual slaughter, are inherently hypocrites. They will in fact eat anything and everything, claiming that their religious practice precludes them from anything that is not kosher. Obesity manifests as a sign of that hypocrisy.

During the nineteenth century, diabetes was seen as a disease of the obese and, in an odd set of associations, the Jew was implicated as obese due to an apparent increased presence of diabetes among Jews. According to one turn-of-the-century specialist, mainly rich Jewish men are fat.[26] But rather than arguing for any inborn metabolic inheritance, he stated that it is the fault of poor diet among the rich—too much rich food and alcohol, this being yet another stereotype of the Jew. And yet, the other side of the coin is amply present.

Jewish scholars reacted in a less than sanguine manner. In the essay on diabetes in the turn-of-the-century *Jewish Encyclopedia*, written by the leading British (Joseph Jacobs) and American (Maurice Fishberg) scholars of the disease of the Jews, there is a clear rejection of the premise that Jews are prone to diabetes for "racial" reasons.[27] They state categorically: "It has also been shown that diabetes is not a racial disease of the Jews." For them diabetes is a disease of "civilization," not of the Jews. As Jews become both emancipated and secularized they come to have all of the diseases of those cultures into which they seem to amalgamate. Thus the dichotomy of Jewish proclivity for as well as immunity against diabetes. "Both of these views," they argue, "(1) that the Jews suffer more frequently from diabetes than other races, and (2) that they are not more often affected—are probably well founded" (554).

It is only a question of the nativity of the Jews: the Jews in Germany, for example, are decidedly more diabetic than those in Russia, England, and France; and the difference of opinion among physicians of experience is simply due to the fact that they usually neglect to consider the question of the nativity of the Jews under consideration. In the United States, where Jews arrive from various countries, diabetes is found to be extremely frequent among the German and Hungarian Jews; while among the Russian Jews it is certainly no more—perhaps it is even less—frequent than among other races. (555)

Diabetes is a disease that becomes evident among Jews as they move from one culture to another, from one world in which they feel to be part of the national identity (Germany) or one where they are alienated (Russia).

Jacobs and Fishberg are forced to confront another theory for the appearance of diabetes among the Jews. Late nineteenth-century anti-Semitism saw the Jews as an essentially "ill" people and labeled the origins of that illness as incest/inbreeding, labeled in the case of the Jews a "consciousness of kind." While the illness that dominated the discourse of the anti-Semitic science was madness (and Jacobs and Fishberg both confront this claim in their own work and elsewhere in *The Jewish Encyclopedia*), diabetes was also attributed to Jewish inbreeding. Its origin too was in the "dangerous" marriages of the Jews, i.e., their refusal to marry beyond the inner group. These marriages were labeled as a criminal activity, even when such "inbreeding" was not consanguineous. In historical terms, writers such as Houston Stewart Chamberlain could comment on the origin of the Jews and its "refreshingly artless expression in the genealogies of the Bible, according to which some of these races owe their origin to incest, while others are descended from harlots."[28] Chamberlain's polemic also appears at the time under the guise of ethnological description. The Jews are described as not only permitting sibling incest (*Geschwisterehe*) historically, but actually practicing it even after they claimed to have forbidden it. The pathological result of such open and/or hidden practices is premature sexual maturity.[29] The various links between deviant forms of sexuality such as sibling incest (or what is understood as sibling incest) and prostitution (the ultimate etiology of mental illness in an age of syphilophobia) placed the Jews and their marriage practices at the center of "biological" concern. And yet there was also a hidden economic rationale in this discussion. For in refusing to marry into the general society, the Jews seemed to be signaling that they were an economic entity, which lived off the general society but did not contribute to it. "Inbreeding" was seen as the origin of the economic hegemony of the Jews and was as poisonous as their sexual activities.

In the literature on diabetes, consanguineous marriages are labeled as more frequent among the Jews than among most other races. It is Jewish practice more than anything that is at the heart of diabetes, according to one group of scholars. "The Jews are the children and grandchildren of town-dwellers," says Charles Bouchard. "In the long run the unfavorable hereditary influences are not rectified for them by the frequent intermarriage of the urban with the country people, as is the case with the rest of the population. The Jews marry exclusively among themselves; first cousins from the paternal or maternal side find no barrier to marriage, and immediately on being born the young Israelite receives the accumulated unfavorable (hereditary) influences, which he further develops during his lifetime, and which tend to the diseases that are generated by disturbed nutrition, particularly diabetes."[30] This Jacobs and Fishberg strongly deny. And yet it is clear in their joint essay in *The Jewish Encyclopedia* on "diathesis" (the "predisposition to certain forms of disease") that they also reject obesity as causal of diabetes. Jews may suffer from "arthritism" under which they "understand a certain group of diseases, usually due to disturbances of the normal metabolism, which manifest themselves primarily as chronic rheumatism and gout, but which also include other morbid processes, such as diabetes, gall-stones, stone in the kidneys, obesity, and some diseases of the skin." But these are "are not racial in the full sense of the word. In the majority of cases they are due to their mode of life, to the fact that Jews are almost exclusively town dwellers, and to the anxieties of their occupations" (574). Obesity remains for them a product of civilization and diabetes is one of its manifestations.

At the beginning of the twentieth century, scientists began to explore the relationship between the predisposition of the Jews for diabetes and the assumed relationship between diabetes and obesity. One physician in 1926 noted that "whereas one in twelve obese Gentiles develops diabetes, no less than one in eight obese Jews develop it. This, it is suggested, is to be explained by the fact that a fat Hebrew is always fatter than a fat Gentile, and that it is the higher grade of obesity which determines the Semitic preponderance in diabetes."[31] The assumption about fat and the "Oriental" race is one that comes to haunt discussions of the meaning of fat.[32] When William H. Sheldon developed his somatotypes in the 1940s, he observed that Jews showed an exaggeration in each of the designated body types. Thus fat Jews are somehow fatter than fat non-Jews.[33] More recent studies of obese Jews look at the complex behavior patterns that occur when religious demands for fasting and the psychological predisposition of the obese come in conflict.[34]

Today, diabetes is not generally considered a Jewish illness. Research now follows the so-called thrifty genotype hypothesis that was suggested in 1964. Simply stated, it has been observed that when sand rats are transferred from a harsh to a benign environment, they gain weight and are hyperglycemic. When one thus measures first-generation groups of immigrants to the United States in the late nineteenth century or in Israel today, there is a substantially higher rate of diabetes. The initial groups, such as the Yemenites who immigrated from a harsh environment, showed an extremely low index of diabetes when they arrived in Israel. This index, however, skyrocketed after just a short time of living in their new environment. Thus, diabetes and obesity seem to be an index of a failure to adapt rapidly to changed surroundings.[35]

And yet fat is still imagined as a Jewish issue, but with a shift in the question of gender. From the 1910s to the present "fat" has become a question for women, rather than the focus of concern about race and masculinity. The columnist David Margolis, writing in the *Los Angeles Jewish Journal* in 2001, observes:

> A lot of people also consider fat a Jewish issue. According to a recent survey in the New York City area, Jewish families consume "almost double" the amount of cake and donuts that non-Jewish families do and more than twice as much diet soda and cottage cheese. A professional in the eating-disorder industry claims that Jews tend to choose food over addictions to other substances. Food is just another drug, after all, the cheapest, most easily available, most socially acceptable mood-altering substance. Is it merely a coincidence that Alcoholics Anonymous was founded by two Christian men, while Overeaters Anonymous was founded by two Jewish women?[36]

The image of the overfed Jew, central to the culture that needed to see the "Oriental" disease of diabetes as an essential aspect of the corrupt Jewish soul, now has a place in American popular culture. Yet, here it is transformed into the body of the Jewish woman, as "fat" in the United States "is a feminist issue."[37]

Fat is a Jewish issue only if being Jewish is, as it seems to be in the *Los Angeles Jewish Journal*, an ethnic rather than a religious category. In a series of essays, Kenneth Ferraro, a medical sociologist, looked at the corollary between religious practice and obesity using data from 1986. In his studies it was clear that "obesity is associated with higher levels of religiosity."[38] Obesity dominated in those parts of the United States that had the highest level of religious practice (and one can add poverty). Southern Baptists in 1998 were the fattest of the Christian denominations, Roman Catholics were at the middle of the scale, and

Jews (and other non-Christians) made up the thin end of his sample. But being Jewish here correlates with membership in congregations, and that correlates with middle class wealth and identity. Ferraro concludes his 1998 article by observing that food and religion provide "a couple of the few pleasures accessible to populations which are economically and politically deprived" (236). Marx was right—religion (and here we can add food) is the opiate of the people. Evidently when Jews are considered as a religious group, rather than as an ethnicity, they are thin enough.

The Literary Image of the Fat Jew

The cultural implications of seeing obesity as a "Jewish" problem (or at least as a problem of the Jews) are echoed in the first attempts to provide a secular, self-critical Jewish literary text. The image of the "fat buddy" in modern literature follows Cervantes's iconic fat man, Sancho Panza, who is a model for the later association of obesity and effeminacy. The fat man in this Jewish continuation of the figure of Sancho Panza does indeed reflect the confusion of gender present in the debates of the nineteenth century and the identification of the "exotic" Jew as the individual at risk from the social stigma of obesity. In the first modern Yiddish novel, Mendele Mocher Seforim's *The Travels and Adventures of Benjamin the Third* (1885), the pairing of the thin and fat protagonists, so well known both from fiction (Quixote and Sancho Panza), as well as from the narratives of overcoming adversity, is repeated with meaningful variations.[39] Here the obese figure is clearly defined with overt attributes ascribed to the feminine in Yiddish popular culture. Mendele's Sancho Panza, Senderel, is "simple-minded, unassuming" (37) and is often the butt of jokes in the synagogue (37). His wife supports him and he takes over the wifely duties in the kitchen. Indeed, he is called Senderel "*die Yiddine*," the housewife (39). Our Quixote, Benjamin, "always found it a pleasure to talk to him. It's quite possible, too, that Benjamin took into consideration Senderel's lack of resistance; Senderel would be bound to agree to his plan" (39). Like Quixote, Benjamin convinces Senderel to leave his family and go with him on an adventure. When they leave home, Senderel is dressed in "a skirt made of calico and woman's headgear" (48). Cervantes's pairing of fat and thin has so pervaded the culture that, by the time of Mendele, there is no longer even any need to evoke body type. It is assumed that Benjamin has a body like that of Cervantes's protagonist and that his Sancho Panza is again "Mr. Gut." But as with the rereading of the Jewish obese body in the diabetes literature of the time, this image of the feminine male has contemporary resonance.

Here the reader is presented with the image of the male Jew as woman. The assumption of nineteenth-century culture was that Jewish males were effeminate. They were not women but a sort of a "third sex," neither male nor female. The image of the male Jew was feminized even in the work of Jewish scientists of the period. Indeed, in expressing the view that the Jews are a single race, the Elberfeld Jewish physician Heinrich Singer commented in 1904 that "in general it is clear in examining the body of the Jew, that the Jew most approaches the body type of the female."[40] Hans Gross, the famed Prague criminologist (and father of the psychoanalyst Otto Gross), commented with ease about the "little, feminine hand of the Jew."[41] These medical views echoed the older anthropological view, which in the mid-1800s the Jewish ethnologist (and rabbi) Adolph Jellinek, stated quite directly: "In the examination of the various races it is clear that some are more masculine, others more feminine. Among the latter the Jews belong, as one of those tribes, which are both more feminine and have come to represent (repräsentieren) the feminine among other peoples. A juxtaposition of the Jew and the woman will persuade the reader of the truth of the ethnographic thesis." Jellinek's physiological proof is the Jew's voice: "Even though I disavow any physiological comparison, let me note that bass voices are much rarer than baritone voices among the Jews."[42] The association of the image of the Jew (here read male Jew) with that of the woman (including the Jewish woman) is one of the most powerful images to be embedded in the arguments about race. And it is the image of the fat woman, the "Oriental," from the late nineteenth century that haunts Mendele's novel. A novel written to critique Eastern European practices and attitudes from the standpoint of the Jewish Enlightenment (Haskalah), its representation of the fat body of Senderel reflects the complex criticism of Haskalah thought on the impact of the ghetto on the Jewish body. Here the line to the question of the diabetic Jew reflecting the nature of his (or her) surroundings is very clear.

Thus Mendele's feminized Senderel seems to be very much in character with Mendele's goals in condemning the mindset of the Eastern European Jews, a mindset that precluded them from seeing the potential for cultural and physical regeneration. And yet the pairing with the emaciated Benjamin provides, within the model provided by Cervantes, an answer that sets these characters off from all other Jews. They are not representative but anomalous, part of the parodic world in which the Jewish body can be displayed because the *Haskalah* offers a mode by which it can be reformed. But the special relationship of the obese body to the feminized male is here used to refute the assumption of the "Oriental" fat boy that haunts the image of the Jew in the West. These paired antiheroes employ the "fat buddy" as a means of characterizing male-male relationships and thus defining masculinity. The literary figure and the autobiographical accounts are cut from the same cultural cloth. Here the links to the post-Pauline images of the decay of the body, specifically the Jewish body, that haunt the French Enlightenment, are reflected in their inclusion in the claims of the Yiddish Enlightenment and its first literary image of the fat Jew. Obesity thus becomes a means of internal social critique in an age when the image of the Jew's body as "Oriental" and thus diseased was central to the debates about race and obesity. The world of Enlightenment fiction echoes the shift in the meaning of the body under Christianity and its secular, scientific successors in the nineteenth century.

In the history of the image of the obese Jew, we can follow how the image of impairment, so important to the definitions of disability, becomes part of an external as well as internal critique of the very notion of handicap. Is a handicap something that is intrinsic or can it be altered and changed? This is at the core of the ideological reading of "race" within the debates about Jewish bodies in the modern age. Disability becomes a way to redefine the nature of Jewish identity as "at risk" and therefore incapable of functioning in the world. Can one change the nature of the Jewish body? Certainly the Jewish Enlighteners and then the Zionists thought that doing so would be a necessary first step in true emancipation. Obesity and diabetes specialists tended to imagine the Jewish body as at risk with various possibilities for change. But the perception remained in all of these representations that there was something in the "essence" of the Jew that was different and abnormal. The obese body represented that difference in complex and often contradictory ways.

NOTES

1. Derek J. Chadwick and Gail Cardew, eds., *The Origins and Consequences of Obesity* (Chichester, UK: John Wiley, 1996).

2. *Americans with Disabilities Act of 1990*, July, 1990, section 2a [law-on-line], http://www.usdoj.gov/crt/ada/pubs/ada.txt (accessed February 6, 2004).

3. *Equal Employment Opportunity Commission Compliance Manual* § 902.2(c)(5), http://www.eeoc.gov/policy/docs/902cm.html (accessed February 6, 2004).

4. *Clemons v. Big Ten Conference*, [1997] WL 89227 (N.D. Ill. 1997), http://www.clccrul.org/2002adeamanual.pdf (accessed February 6, 2004).

5. National Institutes of Health, *Clinical Guidelines on the Identification, Evaluation, and Treatment of Overweight and Obesity in Adults: The Evidence Report* (Bethesda, MD: US Department of Health and Human Services, 1998).

6. Milt Freudenheim, "Employers Focus on Weight as Workplace Health Issue," *New York Times*, September 6, 1999, A15.

7. William R. Miller, ed., *The Addictive Behaviours: Treatment of Alcoholism, Drug Abuse, Smoking, and Obesity* (Oxford: Pergamon Press, 1980); and Jon D. Kassel and Saul Shiffman, "What Can Hunger Teach Us about Drug Craving? A Comparative Analysis of the Two Constructs," *Advances in Behaviour Research and Therapy* 14 (1992): 141–67.

8. "Killjoy Woz Here," *Economist*, March 8, 2003, 75.

9. Ali H. Mokdad et al., "The Spread of the Obesity Epidemic in the United States, 1991–1998," *JAMA* 282, no. 16 (1999): 1519–22.

10. Geoffrey Carr, "The Human Genome," *Economist*, July 1, 2000, 7.

11. H. Tristram Engelhardt, Jr., "The Philosophy of Medicine: A New Endeavor," *Texas Reports on Biology and Medicine* 31, no. 3 (1973): 443–52, 446.

12. Julius Preuss, *Biblical and Talmudic Medicine*, trans. and ed. Fred Rosner (New York: Sanhedrin Press, 1978), 215.

13. *Torah Nebi'im Kethubim: The Holy Scriptures According to the Masoretic Text* (Philadelphia: Jewish Publication Society of America, 1955).

14. Jon L. Berquist, *Controlling Corporeality: The Body and the Household in Ancient Israel* (New Brunswick, NJ: Rutgers University Press, 2002), 34–5.

15. Cited from Daniel Boyarin, "The Great Fat Massacre: Sex, Death, and the Grotesque Body in the Talmud," in *People of the Body: Jews and Judaism from an Embodied Perspective*, ed. Howard Eilberg-Schwartz (Albany: State University of New York Press, 1992), 69–100, 88. I am using Boyarin's rather contemporary translation. The Soncino translation follows: "'Rejoice, my heart! If matters on which thou art doubtful are thus, how much more so those on which thou art certain! I am well assured that neither worms nor decay will have power over thee.' Yet in spite of this, his conscience disquieted him. Thereupon he was given a sleeping draught, taken into a marble chamber, and had his abdomen opened, and basketsful of fat removed from him and placed in the sun during Tammuz and Ab, and yet it did not putrefy. But no fat putrefies!—[True,] no fat putrefies; nevertheless, if it contains red streaks, it does. But here, though it contained red streaks, it did not. Thereupon he applied to himself the verse, My flesh too shall dwell in safety." *The Soncino Talmud*. CD-ROM. Davka Corporation, 2003.

16. *The Holy Bible: Containing the Old and New Testaments in the Authorized King James Version* (New York: Abradale Press, 1970). Subsequent citations from the Christian bible refer to this edition.

17. Samuel S. Kottek, "On Health and Obesity in Talmudic and Midrashic Lore," *Israel Journal of Medical Sciences* 32, no. 6 (1996): 509–10.

18. Maimonides, *Das diätetische Sendschreiben des Maimonides (Rambam) an den Sultan Saladin*, ed. and trans. D. Winternitz (Wien: Braumüller und Seidel, 1843). Compare Fred Rosner, *The Medical Legacy of Moses Maimonides* (Hoboken, NJ: KTAV, 1998).

19. Maimonides, *Medical Writings: The Art of Cure–Extracts from Galen*, ed. and trans. Uriel S. Barzel (Haifa: Maimonides Research Institute, 1992), 175–6.

20. Toby Gelfand, "'Mon Cher Docteur Freud': Charcot's Unpublished Correspondence to Freud, 1888–1893," *Bulletin of the History of Medicine* 62, no. 4 (1988): 563–88, 587.

21. George Henry Lane-Fox Pitt-Rivers, *The Clash of Culture and the Contact of Races* (London: Routledge, 1927), 82.

22. Jean Frumusan, *The Cure of Obesity*, trans. Elaine A. Wood (London: John Bale, 1924), 9.

23. Robert Saundby, "Diabetes mellitus," in *A System of Medicine*, ed. Thomas Clifford Allbutt (London: Macmillan, 1897), 3:167–212, 197–9.

24. William F. Christie, *Obesity: A Practical Handbook for Physicians* (London: William Heinemann, 1937), 31.

25. Max J. Oertel, "Obesity," in *Twentieth Century Practice*, ed. Thomas J. Stedman, vol. 2, *Nutritive Disorders* (New York: William Wood, 1895), 625–728, 647–8.

26. Carl von Noorden, *Die Fettsucht* (Wien: Alfred Hölder, 1910), 63.

27. Joseph Jacobs and Maurice Fishberg, "Diabetes Mellitus," *The Jewish Encyclopedia*, 12 vols. (New York: Funk and Wagnalls, 1905–1926), 4:553–6, 555. Subsequent references are cited parenthetically in the text.

28. Houston Stewart Chamberlain, *Foundations of the Nineteenth Century*, trans. John Lees. 2 vols. (London: John Lane/The Bodley Head, 1913), 1:366.

29. Hans F. K. Günther, *Rassenkunde des jüdischen Volkes* (München: J. F. Lehmann, 1930), 134.

30. Charles Bouchard, *Leçons sur les maladies par ralentissement de la nutrition* (Paris: F. Savy, 1892), quoted in Jacobs and Fishberg, *The Jewish Encyclopedia* 4: 556.

31. Leonard Williams, *Obesity* (London: Humphrey Milford /Oxford University Press, 1926), 52–3.

32. See Jean Leray, *Embonpoint et obésité* (Paris: Masson, 1931), 11–2; William F. Christie, *Surplus Fat and How to Reduce It* (London: William Heinemann, 1927), 1–8, which begins with a long discussion of racial predisposition to fat.

33. William H. Sheldon, Stanley S. Stevens, and William B. Tucker, *The Varieties of Human Physique* (New York: Harper & Brothers, 1940), 221.

34. On fat Jews and fasting Jews see Stanley Schachter, "Who Fasts on Yom Kippur?" in *Emotion, Obesity, and Crime* (New York: Academic Press, 1971), 124–34.

35. Richard M. Goodman, *Genetic Disorders among the Jewish People* (Baltimore: Johns Hopkins, 1979), 337–8, citing Knut Schmidt-Nielsen et al., "Diabetes Mellitus in the Sand Rat Induced by Standard Laboratory Diets," *Science* 143 (1964): 689–90. See also Arthur E. Mourant, Ada C. Kopec, Kazimiera Domaniewska-Sobczak, *The Genetics of the Jews* (Oxford: Clarendon Press, 1978).

36. David Margolis, "Fat: Remember 'Stressed' Spelled Backwards is Desserts," http://www.davidmargolis.com/article.php?id=11 (accessed February 20, 2004).

37. See Susie Orbach, *Fat is a Feminist Issue: The Anti-Diet Guide to Permanent Weight Loss* (New York: Berkley Books, 1979).

38. Kenneth F. Ferraro, "Firm Believers? Religion, Body Weight, and Well-being," *Review of Religious Research* 39, no. 3 (1998): 224–44, 232. Subsequent references are cited parenthetically in the text. See also Cynthia M. Albrecht-Jensen, "Does Religion Influence Adult Health?" *Journal for the Scientific Study of Religion* 30, no. 2 (1991): 193–202; and Jerome Koch, "Religion and Health among Black and White Adults," *Journal for the Scientific Study of Religion* 33, no. 4 (1994): 362–75.

39. Mendele Mocher Seforim, *The Travels and Adventures of Benjamin the Third*, trans. Moshe Spiegel (New York: Schocken Books, 1949). Subsequent references are cited parenthetically in the text. See also Dan Miron, *A Traveler Disguised: A Study in the Rise of Modern Yiddish Fiction in The Nineteenth Century* (New York: Schocken Books, 1973).

40. Heinrich Singer, *Allgemeine und spezielle Krankheitslehre der Juden* (Leipzig: Benno Konegen, 1904), 9, my translation.

41. Hans Gross, *Kriminal-Psychologie* (Leipzig: F.C.W. Vogel, 1905), 121, my translation.

42. Adolph Jellinek, *Der jüdische Stamm: Ethnographische Studien* (Vienna: Herzfeld und Bauer, 1869), 89–90, my translation.

Response to Section I: Dis-ability

Thomas W. Laqueur

These essays move from the particular to the cosmic with vertiginous speed. Tobin Siebers's essay is the most leisurely and, so I thought at first, least threatening; it begins by announcing its subject as passing and moves to an engagement with Eve Kosofsky Sedgwick on the epistemology of the closet—the ways in which the disability closet is, and is not, like that of homosexuality. Almost halfway through we are still more or less securely on well-trod academic ground: What are we to make, Siebers asks, of Joan Riviere's analysis of the intellectually competent woman who puts on a masquerade of feminine flirtation to gain acceptance among her male colleagues? Riviere interprets this behavior as the result of a psychopathology—sadism, rivalry, and desire for supremacy. Siebers, quite rightly, rejects this turn to medicine instead of to politics and finds it particularly offensive in light of the role medicine has played in subjecting women, queers, disabled people, and others. We seem to be in for an analysis of the politics of disability masquerade—of exaggerating, minimizing, displaying, or not displaying some mental or physical feature or some prosthesis associated with them. The narratives that he offers show, he says, how people "manage the stigma of social difference." Fair enough. "Manage" is a general way of including the overtly political along with less-structured negotiations.

But then comes a claim to be reckoned with: disability narratives are urgently important because "they posit a different experience that clashes with how social existence is usually constructed and recorded." They are the basis of identity politics and allow people with different disabilities to tell a story about their common cause. Now here are very big claims—about creating the general from the particular, about the possibility of transcendence—that one could quarrel with for some time.

The other papers move more quickly. In "Meditation, Disability, and Identity," Susan Squier proposes that the new identity shaped by

61

the encounter of disability and meditation can decenter Western medical practice from its exclusively positivist role. This seems a modest claim. One combatant in the struggle for disability civil rights whom Squier quotes argues that just as gay people "automatically understand that gender roles are mostly arbitrary constructions," so "disabled people . . . understand about the illusory nature of our attachment to the body." Another of her narrators seems less sanguine: "[G]reat bravery . . . [the] acceptance of fate, the splendid triumph of spirit over physical self— these were all put-up jobs." Here, the relationship between body and mind (for want of a better word) is up for grabs as urgently as it was in the theology of resurrection and eternal life which so absorbed theologians and poets. Donne worried his whole life about *just* how arbitrary his particular body was to what he hoped would be his resurrected self.

Finally, Sander Gilman's learned account of the putative relationship between fat and Jewishness over the ages and his reading of a novel with a thin protagonist and his fat friend—the Don Quixote buddy narrative—is situated in the effort to understand what counts as healthy and what as ill and provides an entrée into a "wide range of interlocking questions about the cultural construction of the body." It is even more about how we read the bodies around us to make sense of the social world; it is about a physiognomy writ large.

I say this by way of emphasizing the huge ambitions of disability studies and the consequent impossibility of my addressing the larger claims—or even the many smaller ones—of these three essays with the seriousness they deserve. Almost any paragraph demands pages. That being impossible under the circumstances, I will offer instead two short narratives with a message, representative anecdotes with a point if not an argument. My moral comes at the end and not at the beginning where Siebers places his.

Disability, Medicine, and the State

I was at a conference once in the Netherlands where one of my fellow speakers was a Dutch physician whose job it was to define ugliness for the purpose of access to state-sponsored medical care. Her task was to develop criteria that would distinguish those who made demands on public funds for mere cosmetic purposes—those whose noses were not to their liking or wanted some warts removed—and those who were ugly enough to get help from the system. She was trained as a doctor and as an anthropologist and was more than willing to concede the arbitrariness of any possible definition. I do not remember many of her examples of ugliness, but one was that a body be so distorted that clothing size for one part be four sizes different than another. Of course this is arbitrary at almost every level: the standardization of sizes is a recent and bureaucratically established criterion. A mismatch of four sizes has no clearly functional correlative in the body—a person with only a three-size disparity may be as socially stigmatized or impaired in certain tasks as one with four; and the aesthetics of upper- and lower-body proportions vary widely among cultures. In other words, the factor of four is as ontologically indefensible to define one kind of ugliness as is—to use Gilman's example—a body-mass index of more than 100 percent of the norm to define fatness as a disability under the Americans with Disabilities Act.

But such arbitrariness is the product of new demands for distributive justice on the part of the disabled. In both cases—and many others we could all imagine—someone has had to develop categories under which an individual can make claims on the state for medical care, for legal protection, for pensions, for workman's compensation. Someone has to decide by what standards a person is "legally blind" or at what percentage of full capacity they can function or when they are entitled to public funding of medical care or when some condition warrants discrimination. No one, for example, would demand that a restaurateur ignore a communicable disease in a prospective employee, and few would support the right to discriminate on the basis of HIV-positive status. (In fact, with new treatments available in the West, HIV status has moved outside the general orbit of disability.)

Disability and the state of the body are deeply private and deeply cultural matters. But they have also become public to an unprecedented extent, largely through the efforts of the disabled community. Because of this, disability can no longer dwell in the realms of masquerade or personal contemplation. Medicine is a none-too-subtle gatekeeper of disability's public life; its past and to some extent its present cultural biases are ever more apparent. But there have to be experts on the body to do the hard work of producing publicly defensible definitions of disability if the disabled are to make claims on the state or society as well as to ward off discrimination. Medicine proclaims normalcy as well as pathology; it provides the foundation for special exemptions and benefits under certain conditions and for equal treatment under others.

The Personal and the Political

While I was thinking about this response I had a conversation with the director of a large national grass roots organization. Its board is meant to be representative of the country in the sense that it mirrors its diversity in race, gender, geography, sexual orientation, and now also disability status. This poses a problem: Who counts as disabled in this kind of representational politics? I also started thinking about the sign that used to be up in the Paris metro reserving seats for the blind, the lame, invalids of war, and pregnant women. I think that invalids of war are no longer a recognized category, but the others are, I think, still to be given preference and they are certified by the state to be who they claim they are. The signs in most American buses are more general; they ask passengers to give up seats in the front to the disabled and to senior citizens. Sometimes it is clear who is who and what to do. But as I approach sixty, I find myself sometimes calculating whether the latest person to board has a greater claim on the seat than I: yes, maybe a bit older; no, I have bags and he doesn't. Does a deaf person—I know because she is signing—have a greater claim on my seat than I do?

Of course, these are the sorts of calculations we do all the time. We ought to be able to make decisions based upon principles of decency and distributive justice without publicly verifiable certificates of eligibility on the part of people making claims on seats or on early boarding or on being allowed to take a dog into a restaurant. The fact that people often have difficulty doing the right thing left to their own devices makes it necessary to have rules and regulations and criteria that often seem inflexible, silly, or counterproductive. But in general I think it would be a better world if we could do without.

Doing the right thing without regulations and explicit rules, however, depends on trust and truthfulness, on believing that the person with whom we are dealing is who she claims she is. For this to be the case there has to be at least something that is beyond the personal and not a masquerade.

In this sense, perhaps, Tobin Siebers is wrong in maintaining that Dustin Hoffman's performance in *Rain Man* is a form of disability drag in the same sense that his performance in *Tootsie* is what we might call gender drag. I cannot comment on the accuracy of the portrayal of disability. Maybe, to take another example of Siebers's, Sean Penn's performance in *I Am Sam* is, as he claims, a distortion of reality. But drag is not acting. In *Tootsie*, and in drag generally, the game is that we—the audience—know and find pleasure in the constant knowledge that a man is playing a woman or vice versa. Exaggerations of all sorts are constitutive of the genre. But Sean Penn is not in drag playing a retarded person any more than he is in drag playing a condemned rapist/murderer in *Dead Man Walking*. He is playing a role under a set of conventions in which we famously suspend our disbelief and accept him—for the duration of the performance—as someone other than who he is. He is not masquerading; he is acting under the special license of film or theater. If he were playing a retarded person—or a blind or lame person—in a social security office he would be committing fraud. If he were doing disability drag, we would no more treat him as a man with the mental age of seven than we would let a male tennis player in drag enter the women's division of a tournament.

Likewise, we can be nothing but sympathetic with Susan Squier's probing of her own identity, her reflections on whether depression constitutes the grounds for a disabled identity, and whether she should share its role in her life with other people. But the contemplation of subjective identity will not suffice in the many public contexts that these three essays raise or suggest. Identity may "oscillate" for Squier; she may be aware of "a dissolution" of identity and its "impermanence." But if some category called "the depressed" has interests that need to be represented specifically by someone who is, in fact, "depressed"— and likewise for other categories of disability—then there has to be a clear public understanding of what constitutes that category and what its interests are. More generally, there also has to be a theory of why only like can represent like and what exactly constitutes likeness.

I agree with Squier that the discourse of the democratic citizen privileges the "autonomous self." I do not agree that it privileges the intact self precisely because autonomy in this context gives so small a role to the body. Democracy does however assume that we are—or, in any case, are willing to be accountable for—who we appear to be. We do not have to be Rosseauians to believe that willful deployment of masquerade—an open rejection of transparency—is incompatible with a rational and democratic public sphere. And so, while mindful of the dangers of normative state power, we must also be mindful of the antisocial risks of an account of interest and identity that relies largely on subjective criteria and is not open to public debate and scrutiny.

Where the Girls Are:
The Management of Venereal Disease by United States Military Forces in Vietnam

Sue Sun Yom

Introduction

Military health-education films form an intriguing branch of cinema from the standpoint of ideology critique. Inasmuch as they serve military purposes, assisting in the constitution of dependable soldier-subjects (i.e., subjects of the United States military), they are produced and received as unabashed works of propaganda. On the other hand, as films serving purposes of health education, they are yoked to the imperatives of a certain realism, a communication of medical knowledge regarding actual conditions in the field that soldier-viewers can put into effective practice. This contradiction, and the special pressures it exerts on cinematic form, manifest especially graphically in the military sex-education materials of the Vietnam period.

Where the Girls Are—VD in Southeast Asia (hereinafter referred to as *Girls*) was commissioned as a basic sexual-education film just as United States involvement in Vietnam was deepening.[1] Completed as the American military presence reached its height in Southeast Asia, it was first shown to overseas air force personnel and shortly thereafter adopted by the United States Army as well. The film served as an important introduction for new recruits to the culture of Vietnam and was intended to provide realistic medical information for troops on the ground. However, it also demonstrates the mixed impulses at work in the armed forces' efforts to control soldiers' sexual behavior. Its complicated production history and uneven cinematic form provide evidence of the larger mission involved in the making of the ideal American soldier. The film emphasizes a message of psychological and

physical prophylaxis combined with a stereotypical portrayal of Vietnamese women as promiscuous and sexually available. It proceeds on
the basis of numerous formulaic categorizations, most of which reinforced the unequal social and economic power relations between American men and Vietnamese women.

Susan Jeffords, in a study of masculinization and representation of
the Vietnam War, argues that "an important way to read the war,
perhaps the most significant way when we think about war itself, is as
a construction of gendered interests." In her discussion, Jeffords points
out that "patterns of power relations established in the domination of
men over women are employed to set systems of dominance over other
groups as well."[2] In the history of Western cinema, visual techniques
have proven a durable means of constructing gendered patterns of
dominance. In *Girls*, the male soldier's dominance over an invented
version of Vietnam is emphasized by a cinematic vocabulary that
reinforces the centrality of the visiting soldier over the exotic and
feminized world he encounters. This willfully disconnected fantasy of
visual consumption reinscribes traditional gender relations in an international context. The power of these scenes draws upon a long history
of cinematic reification of a passive and sexualized female body.[3]

Relying on these familiar patterns, *Girls* reenacts the customary
power structure of traditional gender relations in Western cinema
within the context of Vietnam. This essay examines the effects of this
ideological backdrop on the deployment of sexual-health policy. As in
other wars, military efforts to address sexually transmitted disease
during the Vietnam War were complicated by overlapping and competing interests aimed at enforcing a certain visual and psychological
stereotype of American masculinity and soldiery. What makes *Girls*
unique is its contemporary setting in the international and interracial
context of Vietnam in the early 1970s, which is exploited to dramatic
effect throughout the film. The particular anxieties associated with
America's long and frustrating history of military involvement in
Vietnam are transmitted, in part, through a strategy of prophylactic
venereal-disease management based on instilling fear of Vietnam—and
Vietnamese women—in the minds of American soldiers.

Addressing VD

Although the official policy of the United States Department of
Defense has always been "to suppress prostitution whenever possible,"

by the time of the Vietnam War, sexual adventure with foreign women was regarded by most military leaders as an inevitable part of the modern military experience.[4] The 1960s saw a general relaxation of American societal mores governing sexuality, with concomitant effects on the attitude of the personnel who served in the United States military. The sexual revolution in the United States, facilitated by the availability of oral contraception after 1965, contributed to higher rates of premarital sex and venereal infection, even as federal funding for venereal-disease control was repeatedly reduced over the course of the 1950s and consistently underfunded in the 1960s and 1970s.[5] As a result, the relative timidity of most military-sponsored, World War II-era, sex-education campaigns gave way to increasingly frank materials capable of reaching a jaded postwar population. Growing numbers of women overseas worked within an international, commercially sponsored prostitution industry tailored to the tastes of American military personnel.[6] Senior military officials not only faced the continuing drain of debilitated soldiers affected by venereal illness but also contended with the additional burden of political conflict with host countries over a flourishing internationalized prostitution industry.

In earlier wars, sexual-education materials focused on the importance of military camaraderie and loyalty to the "small group" of one's fellow soldiers, with the conclusion that contracting venereal disease was a form of laziness and irresponsibility that led to less safety and more work for others.[7] However, in the Vietnam era, sexual behavior had come to be regarded as a sphere of personal autonomy over which the military held very little rightful authority. The psychological disillusionment of the military experience in late-era Vietnam, exacerbated by lagging support from civilian sectors, encouraged pessimism and fatalism among the rank-and-file, resulting in an increased use of sex and narcotics.[8] In addition, the availability of antibiotics contributed to a sentiment widely held throughout the United States that venereal disease was curable and, at its worst, a temporary inconvenience, even though antibiotic-resistant gonorrhea was a matter of increasing medical concern in Vietnam.[9]

In this setting, *Girls* was considered an "urgent requirement" and an "urgent need" by United States Air Force headquarters in July 1968.[10] During a trip to Southeast Asia, Air Force Secretary Harold Brown was "shocked as to the high VD rates" and communicated this to United States Defense Secretary Clark Clifford, who in turn, made sure that General John P. McConnell, the air force chief of staff, "for a few days was up to his 'ears in VD.'"[11] A supervising project officer warned that if film production did not proceed, "The capability of the overseas command to fulfill its mission could be jeopardized without adequate indoctrination and education in health subjects."[12] Such recommendations guaranteed immediate attention. McConnell directed the Air Force Medical Service "to get, ASAP, a realistic film in our indoctrination programs," an order that was passed from headquarters to the Norton Air Force Base's Aerospace Audio-Visual Service.[13] *Girls* was released in early 1969 for use among air force personnel and was subsequently adopted by the United States Army in Vietnam (USARV).[14] It was intended to comprise the major component of a venereal-disease prevention session and was accompanied by a sheet of teaching and talking points to introduce and discuss the film. The working title for the project was *VD in SEA* (an abbreviation for Venereal Disease in Southeast Asia), until the "more appropriate and interesting title" of *Where the Girls Are* was added a few weeks later, heralding the project's turn from newsreel or documentary toward feature film.[15] The only major feature production issued by the United States armed services about this topic during the Vietnam War, the film was striking enough to be sold at military retail outlets decades after the war ended.[16] *Girls* was produced "to inform officers and airmen on types and prevalence of venereal disease in Southeast Asia." It was "designed to motivate AF [air force] personnel in avoiding the hazards and tragedies of becoming a victim." The film would emphasize "prevention rather than cure" and be "dramatic enough to provide strong motivation."[17]

In its finished form, *Girls* follows the naïve and clean-cut young air force sergeant, Peter A. Collins, through the shock of arrival for his first tour of duty in Vietnam. In his first few days, Pete makes the acquaintance of his commanding officer, J. P. Hall, an experienced veteran of the Korean War, as well as Ernie King, a fellow soldier whose major recreational activity is to frequent Vietnamese sex-entertainment venues. In a segment highly reminiscent of the lecture-style venereal-disease films used by the military in earlier wars, an educational lecture is shown in which Pete and his fellow soldiers are taught the importance of avoiding sexually transmitted diseases and are counseled to abstain from sex or use a condom with local women. At first, Pete maintains his loyalty to his hometown sweetheart, Julie, and he writes letters to her frequently. But after a long time of receiving no reply, he goes out with Ernie King to a bar and then a massage parlor. Soon afterwards, Pete is diagnosed with gonorrhea. He is shown in line outside the medical office next to Ernie King, who has also come for treatment. The base medical officer scolds King and warns him, in particular, of the danger of long-term urinary sequelae from repeated infection. He also expresses dismay that Pete has not taken the precaution of using condoms and counsels him that abstinence is the only sure method to prevent infection. Chastened, Pete returns to work, and soon thereafter, receives a large packet of letters from Julie that had been delayed in the mail. Pete is relieved and does well until he goes on a rest and recuperation (R&R) visit, where he becomes lonely. He initiates a relationship with another Asian woman during his stay. Pete then returns to his base and is informed that his father has fallen ill. He is given leave to fly home, and there he reunites with Julie. During a romantic interlude, they decide to get married. Unfortunately, after undergoing premarital testing for the marriage license, Pete is found to have syphilis. Furthermore, he has to tell Julie that he may have infected her. The film ends on a somber note, with Pete's mournful intonation, "You can't promise a girl like Julie you'll be true to her and show up with a case of syphilis."

The Theater of Asia

From its opening sequence, *Girls* emphasizes the difference in the two major environments—the United States and Asia—that Pete navigates throughout the film. The first scenes convey a relaxed, secure intimacy captured in close-up shots of Julie and Pete kissing, but these are abruptly swept from the screen, signifying the brusque cut to an inscrutable and dangerous place. At that point, Sergeant Peter A. Collins, air force communications specialist and central narrator of the film, begins a remorseful retrospective. "They shipped me," he says sadly, "to Southeast Asia." The dissonant twang of an Oriental-style musical instrument punctuates Pete's fate. A glaringly bright foreign tarmac, with a plane taxiing in for the landing, is established as the entry to a new stage of action. Pete and J. P. Hall, his commanding sergeant, deplane and survey a flat, sunny airfield. A title rolls down, reading, "The United States Air Force presents," at which point, an Asian shopkeeper appears and unfurls a rattan blind, which metamorphoses into another full-screen film title. The words "Where the Girls Are" appear in bamboo-style lettering on the rattan background, while to the right appears a caricatured sketch of the back of a topless Asian entertainer, clad only in a black-and-white thonglike undergarment.

This special effect was added at the request of air force reviewers. Instead of using a plain opening title, the project supervisor opted to "shoot the title live using a rattan rolled outdoor screen—dropped by an Oriental proprietor in front of his establishment."[18] The shopkeeper's screen, rolling down like a theater curtain, establishes Southeast Asia as an unreal configuration of spectacle and shopping mall—a display of the sheer exoticism of the Asian continent, a feast of the senses, a theatrical scene. Vietnam, as Trinh Minh-ha has observed, is particularly a place to be watched, a place that exists as a spectacle for the West.[19] Or, in the terms laid out by Johannes Fabian, the concept of Otherness, as separate from oneself, has often been invented by imagining an ahistorical "topos of travel" distanced through relationships of time and space.[20] In the context of this film, Pete's displacement signifies the convergence of combat and the sex-entertainment business. He reports for life-threatening duty in a place of international conflict, but this theater of war is skillfully elided with the theater of Asia, represented by the image of the scantily clad cartoon woman.

Over the course of the Korean and Vietnam Wars, Southeast Asia was transformed into a marketplace that specialized in the peddling of sex. Asian governments formally insisted on the dignity of their women, mostly due to discontent among traditionalist constituents disturbed by the large number of Asian women involved with American men.[21] Nonetheless, the reality was that commercial interests proved irresistible influences, not only over the majority of the local populace but also over a government structure infiltrated by investors and profiteers. At the time when the armistice ending the Korean War was signed, the United States had thirty-seven thousand troops on ninety-nine bases and installations in South Korea, and twenty-seven thousand women were living in the areas around the bases.[22] As instability escalated in the mid-1950s, American advisors began reshaping the firepower and supply services of the southern Vietnamese army, and in 1962, tens of thousands more American troops entered the Asian theater.[23] Almost twice as many Americans, about 3.4 million, served in Vietnam as in World War I.[24] The typical soldier had more cash on hand than most Vietnamese saw in a year.

In Saigon, the intended major setting of *Girls*, two notable early landmarks in the rise of the nighttime entertainment industry were the overthrow of the Ngo Dinh Diem government in 1963 and the influx of stationed American troops. According to a State Department analysis, Diem's regime had exercised an uncompromising attitude toward Saigon's nightlife. After 1963, however, an atmosphere of financial opportunism took hold and was backed by "several ranking military officers who were to have financial interests in the new entertainment spots." Growth continued steadily until 1965, when an influx of thirty thousand American troops into the Saigon metropolitan area "brought undreamed of opportunities." Several hundred other American troops came monthly to Saigon on brief R&R stays. According to this analysis, "Saigon's impresarios rose to the challenge," licensing bars, nightclubs, cabarets, hotels, and restaurants. In 1965–6, the United States Military Assistance Command, Vietnam (MACV) declared a ban on R&R leaves in Saigon in an attempt to stem the rising tide of nighttime activity, but by that time, a newly arriving population of American civilian contractors were providing a new base of customers for this business sector.[25]

In early 1966, three years before *Girls* was issued, Saigon contained over one thousand bars, over one hundred nightclubs, and at least thirty cabarets. These statistics only represented the businesses registered with the city. The combined tax on these establishments comprised 14 percent of the city's annual revenue. An estimated twenty-five thousand women worked as bar girls, while nightclub and bar service employees numbered over twenty thousand. By the beginning of 1966, MACV had succeeded in redeployment efforts so that only twelve thousand servicemen were permanently stationed in Saigon. At the end of 1967, a survey by the American Embassy in Saigon indicated that Maxim's, the most expensive nightclub in Saigon, had connections to General Nguyen Ngoc Loan, the National Police chief, and that the Queen Bee, a club second only to Maxim's, was owned by the family of Tran Van Tuat, a former USARV lieutenant.[26] In the end, the report remarked upon "a reluctance to ruin what is to many Saigonese a first-rate business, the entertainment sector" and concluded that despite efforts to control its growth, "Saigon's night life apparently will continue to thrive in one form or another."[27]

In 1967, five hundred thousand troops were in Vietnam and another four hundred thousand were stationed in the nearby northeastern provinces of Thailand.[28] In 1969, at the time *Girls* was finally ready for release, United States military presence in Asia was at its height, and troops in Vietnam alone numbered about five hundred and fifty thousand. An estimated several hundred thousand women had passed through the entertainment industry.[29] In fact, in the 1960s, the Republic of South Vietnam, Thailand, Hong Kong, and the Philippines signed agreements, facilitated and sometimes financed by members of the military elite within their respective countries, to provide services at R&R centers for American military and aid personnel. Between 1967 and 1970, spending by United States military personnel on R&R leave in Thailand grew from $5 million to around $20 million. In this context,

Pete's exploration of the sex trade in *Girls* reflects the growing business of servicing American soldiers overseas. The theater of war in Southeast Asia intimately converged with the theater of sexual entertainment, and both exercised a profound effect on the experience of the American soldier serving in Vietnam.

Prostitution in the Imagination of Asia

The United States military's approach to venereal-disease education during the two world wars had been to emphasize the improper sexual behavior, avarice, and uncleanliness of non-American women.[30] *Girls* proceeded on a similar basis in enacting a comparable characterization of the women of Vietnam. Much as France had been considered a highly sexualized and perverse culture in the sexual-education materials of World War I, Vietnam was thought to be an exotic place of wanton women for sale at a cheap price. As noted by its makers, *Girls* was designed so that it "ESTABLISHES the Southeast Asian scene and its differing and more permissive atmosphere with respect to the sexual behavior of American servicemen."[31]

Prostitution was a fertile metaphor that infiltrated all areas of commercial life in Vietnam. In international political terms, it also signified a humiliating dependency. For example, a 1967 embassy report noted the comments of a French business resident of Saigon, who stated, "Saigon's heavy industry is prostitution to all kinds of rich people, whether they are foreigners or not." The report tendered the astute analysis that "the word 'prostitution' [signifies] an alleged desire among Vietnamese to acquire a better life for themselves regardless of the means to be used."[32] The impression that the Vietnamese people were prostituted or desired to prostitute themselves was a metaphoric screen that heavily influenced relationships between Vietnam and the West. As dissipated serviceman Ernie King calls it in the film, Vietnam represented "sensuous southeast Asia, land of the slope-eyed broads and scented baths."[33]

Yet prostitution was a shameful affair for the local populace and therefore only reluctantly acknowledged by Asian governments.[34] Discussion of the topic was so charged an issue that determining the filming location of *Girls* evolved into a series of international negotiations requiring considerable finesse.[35] At one point, the filmmakers hoped to shoot footage off-base in Naha City, Okinawa, but a memorandum in November 1968 laid out the difficulties: "Because of the nature of the film, we cannot shoot covertly—everything must be approved, and the shooting will be overt. The only place where we could be sure of foreign Government approval is Saigon, and to go to Saigon with a commercial crew and actors poses other problems that might be restricting." In the end, it was deemed diplomatically unfeasible to film anywhere in Asia except on the American-governed territory of the air force bases themselves.[36]

Asian governments did not wish to have their territories documented on film as havens for prostitution, especially from the point of view of an American military production. In truth, the Asian countries where Pete travels serve only as backdrops to the moral crisis he experiences. Pete's story becomes that of the perils of "the psychic and ethical dislocation of young men," and the sea of suggestive sights and sounds culled from the Asian surround functions as a reflection of Pete's interior psychological landscape.[37] Explaining or portraying the appalling conditions of prostitution in Asia is not a priority; demonstrating Pete's mistaken decision-making process is.

A draft of the film script describes the opening montage as follows:

> Women of Southeast Asia on the streets of the city—A series of wild shots—The camera in motion—Shots intercut to give a psychedelic [sic] effect of various parts of anatomy in motion—but this should be subtle, suggestive, very Oriental—vague, shifting movements of a leg, a mouth, a hand, an arm, a face, eyes, breasts, heads, backs, bellies, feet, etc. Intercut to the rhythm of the music.[38]

Shots of Asian women flash on-screen at a breakneck pace. The emphasis is upon the women's interactions with American soldiers. A long shot shows an "Oriental girl" who speaks with an airman in fatigues; she is wearing a miniskirt.[39] A rapid cut switches to another girl speaking to an airman. A girl waves and playfully slaps a serviceman, as the camera dollies in to a closer angle. The camera pans, showing the lower bodies of two girls seated on a motor bike. Two girls with their arms around each other walk forward, offering a tightly focused shot of their buttocks. A skirt is pulled up, or a thigh is stroked, interspersed with large close-ups of women smiling. Abruptly spliced and varied in subject, shot length, and angle, this series provides a rapid transition into a dizzying selection of exotic, interchangeable body parts. "Oriental" music adds to the unfamiliarity of the scene.

The street montage was constructed by military filmmakers from assembled stock shots commissioned especially for this film.[40] These were supplied from footage procured by the 1350th motion picture squadron, in consultation with the leadership of other air force film units and the contracted film director. Instructions for film production support were sent in December 1968 from AAVS headquarters to a camera unit assigned to shoot footage at Tan Son Nhut Air Force Base and in downtown Saigon. The assignment was labeled "most important" and the unit commander was directed "to give this assignment earliest possible support with best people available." One of the three sections of the list of requested scenes specified shots of downtown Saigon, including "closer shots of Drinking Parlors, Movie house, public market and foreign looking signs and objects." Of particular interest were "street scenes, close shots of signs over businesses, particularly of a steam bath parlor," and "Targets of Opportunity to feature, as close as possible, some of the more attractive features of the local girls." These shots were to be taken in "DAY & NIGHT." The instruction was to maximize the visual interest of the scenes: "These should, if possible, feature the parts of the anatomy in motion which men will turn their heads to watch."[41] Another, later memo from a USAF film library referenced available "stock footage of downtown Saigon showing Flea Market, Steam Bath, tourist attractions and girls."[42] It was intended that Saigon would be presented as a collection of foreign objects, tourist sites, and sexual-entertainment options—presenting a somewhat fantastical view of Vietnamese life as it was thought to be perceived by the American soldier.

These montages link Pete's fictional adventures in the film to the construction of a seductive world of Asian women that surrounds the soldier viewer in the audience—a thrilling, consumerist simulacrum of Saigon's presumed reality. Although most of the women filmed for these montages were surely not prostitutes, nevertheless it is the visual conglomeration of Asian women's bodies that will seduce Pete, called "the victim" in the script, to commit a form of adultery.[43] The overwhelming plentitude and variety of the bodies that greet Pete's arrival in Asia—spectacular, fascinating, and so obviously different from anything in his previous experience—are intended to channel an unmediated visual shock to the spectator, establishing that Pete's mistake is less willful than inevitable.

Moreover, the camera's obsessive examination of these women, in a variety of poses and angles, gives life to Pete's growing fascination, initiating anxiety and generating desire. These montages, a suspension in a fantasy world replete with sexual overtones, function, as described by Linda Williams, to facilitate the movement from "equilibrium to disequilibrium and back," with disequilibrium configured as the "process of desire itself and the various blockages to its fulfillment."[44] Williams notes that the function of sex scenes in a pornographic feature are multivalent; they act as moments of pleasure that may be gratifying either to viewers or to the characters, statements or restatement of sexual conflicts, or resolutions of conflicts in either the narrative or other sex scenes.[45] Thus these sexual montages are able to contain the multiple burdens of fantasy, plot dissociation, and spectatorial desire that infuse their watching. The montages channel the film's fundamentally ambivalent approach to sexual activity and sexual desire, derived from the simultaneous, contradictory economies created by the formal prohibition of sexual relations with foreign women and the striking visual consumption of sexual pleasure promoted by the aesthetics of the film. This dilemma harkens back to similar debates dating from World War II which characterized the publication of sexual-education materials as overly arousing or of a nature that would inspire an unsafe interest in sexual activity.[46] *Girls* embodies the inherently contradictory nature of the military's approach to sexual-health management, which remained confined to an absolutist morality—with abstinence the most preferred mode of prevention—that was fatally divorced from the realities of soldiers' experiences.

Reality and Representation

Obtaining the correct military look on-screen required significant effort by the filmmakers. The principal actors had begun the filming with sideburns and long hair, but as one memorandum on the subject contended, "Some of the professional actors in the role of Air Force enlisted personnel in Southeast Asia did not reflect the proper Air Force image." The actors' sideburns and long hair were at first approved by the USAF's supervising producer, because "the actor's appearance (haircut, sideburns, moustache) truly reflected typical GIs ['general issue' soldiers] in SEA." However, the unit chief and section chief insisted that "when Air Force personnel are depicted on the screen, they should insofar as possible represent the ideal Air Force image."[47] Shooting at Norton AFB was temporarily cancelled, and the actors were given appropriate haircuts and shaving for "re-accomplishment of the photography," at an estimated cost to the air force of over one fourth of the entire film budget.[48] While unable to regulate troops' actual appearance, commanders demanded an on-screen portrayal of the ideal soldier.

Conflict over the proper military haircut arose from the perception of a lack of discipline among enlisted troops. Proper appearance became a flashpoint that consolidated commanders' frustration over the inadequacy of established training techniques in the face of potent social influences encouraging individualism and anti-institutional rebellion. The makers of *Girls* deliberately chose to present an idealization of the clean-cut, upstanding military appearance. All of Pete's commanders, who attempt to warn him away from unhealthy sexual habits, have relatively short, military-style haircuts. On the other hand, the character of Ernie King, who initiates Pete into the seamy nightlife of Saigon, sports an unkempt, shaggy haircut and a moustache. King's appearance is all the more noticeable in the film among the band of newly shaven actors. King becomes the engineer of Pete's initial descent into the Asian sex world. His unwholesome influence on the naïve Collins bears out the early visual indices of his bad military character.

In truth, the realities of daily life for the average soldier in Vietnam did not match the requirements or the ideals of military policy. In few arenas was this as annoying to commanders as in the matter of sexual-health regulation. An influential internal summary of the military's preventive medicine policy in 1971 stated, "[Preventive-medicine] policy adheres to that of the Army. Prostitution will be suppressed." The summary recommended that areas populated by prostitutes or establishments with a high VD rate be placed off-limits, and if not, that the military police be allowed to "work with the local civil officials to minimize the normal accompanying incidents of assault, drunkenness, AWOL, etc."[49] Despite reiterations of official policy, however, army officials expressed extreme frustration at their inability to limit their troops' exposure to prostitution. A high-ranking colonel complained in 1971, "Of all troop stations prostitution is highest in Vietnam and Korea. It runs wild out there." He added, "Suppression is our policy. If we can do it suppression is best. Unfortunately, in some areas we just can't do it. . . . We have enough trouble regulating haircuts let alone their sex habits."[50] In contrast to the idealization of the soldier that was represented in *Girls*, military commanders accepted multiple forms of compromise with their troops over issues of appearance and sexual behavior.

For decades, the decision to promote the use of condoms had been one of the most contentious issues in military health policy, and the influence of this debate is clearly present in *Girls*. Condoms were not offered to soldiers until World War II, when they were first distributed in what were called "pro kits." Because the concept of prophylaxis was so controversial, condoms were euphemistically labeled a form of "early treatment."[51] Many health officials expressed concern that the use of condom prophylaxis would encourage soldiers to be more promiscuous.[52] However, by the time of the Vietnam War, condoms were well accepted as a necessary compromise to protect the health of men serving overseas. Prevention and prophylaxis became military health strategies that were promoted with almost as much enthusiasm as celibacy. However, even with the use of condoms, venereal-disease incidence rates continued to skyrocket among troops stationed in Asia. *Girls* was part of an ongoing effort to control these escalating rates of disease. Yet the film addresses the topic of condoms only in the most general of terms, during an initial lecture delivered by a health officer and during a subsequent medical examination when Pete learns he is infected. No instruction about condom use or efficacy is provided. Furthermore, the sexualization of Vietnamese women is temporally and conceptually separate from the few sections of the film where condoms are mentioned. The realities of the military's compromise position regarding condom use and prophylaxis are obscured in favor of a stupefying vision of Vietnam as a place where sex is a female commodity.

That Pete and the women he encounters seem like pornographic caricatures is no accident. The figures in *Girls* operate as stand-ins that represent prototypical agents in the interaction of male American soldiers and Vietnamese women. Just as Pete is an artificial and unreal presence, so too are the Vietnamese women he encounters. Both were created from an imaginative perspective of Vietnam that ignored details. Pete is never shown in a sexual position with a Vietnamese woman, and the specific details of the sex act and prophylaxis strategies are not described in the film. The prostitutes in the film appear as aggregated sexual phantoms, without names, personal histories, or spoken dialogue. They are simply visual representations of the unpredictable dangers posed to American servicemen abroad.

In fact, reality was so little a concern in the making of the film that the prostitutes in the film were, for the most part, not Vietnamese. For instance, the script called for Pete and King to solidify their friendship by visiting a bar, at which point a second sensational montage was to be placed. Because of the denial to film overseas, the shots used for this bar montage were filmed in a rented nightclub in Los Angeles, California. The sets were required to "simulate downtown Saigon, back streets, bars, bath houses, streets and bordellos" but were assembled "on location in the general Los Angeles Chinese and Japanese communities." The nightclub was arranged to simulate an "Oriental bar."[53] American women of Chinese and Japanese ancestry were hired to play the roles of Vietnamese bar girls. Instead of wearing the layered Vietnamese *ao dai*, several of the actresses dressed in high-necked silk *qi pao* cut in the Chinese style, but this was sufficient in the race-based logic of this film to represent the rapacious, exotic Vietnamese woman. In this scene, jarring music plays in the background while blurred and distorted shots of Asian women are shown kissing the two American soldiers, smiling, licking their lips, raising their skirts, and caressing their own thighs. Pete drinks heavily and is shown laughing uncontrollably. Later that night he will end up, with King, at a massage session in an upstairs sauna bath. This episode will result in Pete's initial infection with gonorrhea.

This representation of American-Vietnamese relations enacts a slippage that tends to feminize Vietnam in relation to the United States. That is, this staging enacts a displacement of the actual relationship of two countries by focusing exclusively on a preexisting ideological structure defined by gender difference. American masculinity is literally and symbolically configured in the person of Pete Collins. No Vietnamese males are shown except for the lone elderly shopkeeper at the beginning of the film; the country is represented primarily by its women, despite the fact that Vietnamese men had a controlling interest in and profited substantially from the prostitution industry. Vietnam, or more generally, Asia, is symbolically associated with femininity. In addition, the dramatization of the process of spectacle is enacted as a self-perpetuating, avaricious consumerism. Imaginative configurations of what Vietnamese women might offer provide the fuel that supplies the Vietnamese sex market, but the film simultaneously converts this desire to deprivation amidst plentitude. The portrayal of these women as purely sexual beings creates a shopping mall-style fantasy that obscures the cash-driven reality of the illicit market funded by the labor of these women. Thus *Girls* both reflects and elaborates upon a fantasy of Vietnam that is based on personal pleasure, and which models this pleasure-seeking economy on a world in which only American men and Vietnamese women exist.

The gap between the reality of the soldier-financed sex industry in Southeast Asia versus the expectations of military policy ran parallel to the difference between the idealized visual packaging of the clean-shaven Pete and the actual appearance and behavior of the typical soldier. That is, the fundamental problem with *Girls's* visual reproduction of the sexual experience in Asia is that it was predicated on a set of simplistic, conceptually narrow character development parameters. Pete represents a soldier figure that is far removed from the stressful, debilitating, and dehumanizing reality of life in Vietnam, just as the women in the film represent a version of Vietnamese prostitution that is far removed from the disgrace, isolation, and sexual exploitation that characterized their experience. The soldier–prostitute relationship was not isolated from the socioeconomic context of Vietnam itself, nor was it independent of the gendered power structure in Vietnamese society, which allowed prostitution to flourish as a viable money-making option for male pimps able to exploit impoverished Vietnamese women with promises of a better livelihood. Likewise, the fact of the military's compromise with promiscuity, exemplified by widespread distribution of condoms and other sanctioned mechanisms that enabled sex-trade activities near military stations, was downplayed in *Girls* in favor of a dramatized set of consequences that instilled both fear and fascination with Vietnamese women, at the expense of a more nuanced or specific discussion that might have provided deeper and more lasting benefit.

Home and Family

In the concluding segment of the film, Pete returns home after having served in Vietnam for several months. He and Julie hold hands as they walk through the entrance of the hospital where Pete's father has been admitted. The deep immersion into the Vietnamese experience that has characterized the film fades away into an iconic image of suburban American bliss. This distant, proper vision of Julie, the dutiful girlfriend, stands in contrast to the drenching, sensational close-ups that lent the montages of Asian women such compelling power. Despite the opening scenes earlier in the film documenting Julie's sexual activities with Pete, Julie now appears as the opposite of Pete's Asian paramours, or in the words of the filmmakers, she becomes "the girl in all the ads."[54] Pete's future is immutably tied to his relationship with Julie.[55] Thus the film reasserts the virtue of the American girl. To have surrendered to the temptations confronting the military man in Asia is a stain not only on Pete's own honor but on that of his woman waiting at home. The film reasserts a highly conservative vision of domesticity in order to buttress its case against involvement with Vietnamese women.

The opposition between Julie and the women of Asia is structurally built into the film's soundtrack. The production contractor, Jerry Warner, added "a 'Julie' theme at those points where Julie was present either actually or in thought" and "an Oriental 'threat' theme over scenes where it was appropriate to the action, including the scene near the end where the Doctor informs [Pete] of his [syphilitic] condition."[56] The Oriental threat theme, a tinkling melody interspersed with a hollow percussive sound, cuts in for a few seconds after the doctor speaks the diagnosis. As Pete sits in shock and then walks out to the waiting room, he is accompanied by the Julie theme, a wistful flute melody that echoes itself as it weaves in and out of a central, repeating motif.

In the finished film, the final shot is of Julie's face as she stares up at Pete, whose last monologue has just ended: "Sure they give you shots and tell you you're okay, but you can't promise a girl like Julie you'll be true to her and show up with a case of syphilis." In the original script, the writer called for Pete's monologue to run longer, with the lines: "Maybe, if two people love each other enough, they can forget. But I don't think Julie ever will really forget." This section of the monologue, however, was removed "to eliminate the harsh wording which was not typical of our central character."[57] The possibility of return to Julie had to be left open for the soldier in the audience. Thus the prevention of venereal disease depends on a highly traditional specification of the nature of home, fidelity, and chastity; and the narrative logic depends on the presence of the waiting, forgiving American woman.

Conclusion

In one conversation in *Girls*, Ernie King tells Pete, "I mean, this is the greatest place in the world. You don't have to know where the girls are. You don't even have to ask." What King's assertion fails to note is that prostitution did indeed exist at a considerable effort. International sex work was a form of trade that depended on the American dollar and was supported by a complex set of ideological constructions that regarded another country's women as consumerist items for Americans and which, in the converse, employed the possibility of return to American women as a reason to avoid deeply informed or permanent involvement in Vietnam. *Girls*'s presentation of the experience of sexual disease as a personal choice managed by the individual soldier ignored the fact of the complex ideological interdependence of the United States' military policies and the Vietnamese sex industry.

After the withdrawal of American troops, the sex industry in Vietnam gradually dwindled. For instance, in Danang, where there had been a "flourishing bar trade" numbering in the dozens of establishments, there were only five in late 1973, employing only about three hundred bar girls. A State Department report observed that, of the 10 percent of women who continued to work as prostitutes in Danang:

> [L]ife is tough. Lean economic conditions now grip Danang and other MR [metropolitan region]/metropolitan areas. There are few Americans left to patronize bars and pleasure houses. Few Vietnamese have enough money to splurge on a regular basis. Historically, prostitutes are at the bottom rank of the social ladder. Those who have lived with Americans, and particularly those with American [Amerasian] children, are scorned as "spoiled."[58]

Children of American soldiers born to Vietnamese women were considered "family blemishes" or "social inferiors" and faced lives of poverty, servitude, and sexual and financial exploitation.[59] Meanwhile, the establishment of prostitution in other Asian countries became the ongoing legacy of military occupation. In peripheral countries such as Thailand and the Philippines, sex tourism did continue after the American withdrawal of troops from Vietnam. Dependent on the revenue generated by sex-entertainment centers, these surrounding countries continued to court the remaining American soldiers permanently stationed in South Korea, as well as civilians from Europe, Japan, and the United States. In the early 1980s, estimates were that in Bangkok there were 119 massage parlors, 119 barbershops-cum-massage parlors and teahouses, 97 nightclubs, 248 disguised brothels, and 394 disco/restaurants, all selling sexual companionship.[60]

The dynamics addressed in *Girls*—the continuous sexual availability of the Asian women in the film, the erosion of military discipline in the face of powerful sexual fantasy, and the inability to address the rudimentary realities of sex with prostitutes—were, in point of fact, the very constructions undergirding and eliding the complex association between the presence of the American military and the subsequent financing and development of Asia's sexual-entertainment industries. In the face of growing antiwar and antimilitary sentiment, *Girls* produced a vision of Southeast Asia that was far removed from the deadly combat that threatened the life of the ordinary soldier. Instead, Asia was transformed into a consumerist, feminized paradise characterized by sexual pleasure—a place to be carefully managed and generally avoided, much like venereal infection itself. This was an ideology realized in vivid visual terms, translated via imagery associated with male dominance and American political power.

The confused message of *Girls* embodied the contradictions of United States military policy in Asia, which on the one hand recommended the formal elimination of prostitution and yet on the other acceded to only certain of its practical demands. Intense pressure from local Asian governments and home communities required that the military adhere to a formal policy of no-tolerance for prostitution. Yet, in indoctrinating its soldiers in the vocabulary and imagery of a fundamentally exploitative sex trade, the military acted in de facto support of a sex industry that victimized Southeast Asian women. As political theorist Cynthia Enloe has postulated, the circumstances of post–World War II prostitution in Asia were not haphazard but required bureaucracies, ideologies, and representations, however subtly expressed, to carry them out. Enloe argues for a denaturalization of this relationship to demonstrate that decisions and actions by both American and foreign governments enabled the existence of the sex trade as an industry.[61]

Thus *Girls* claims realism as its purpose while refusing to confront the actual conditions of the sex trade. The emphasis of military commanders that the film be "realistic," a request meant to differentiate this production from the out-of-date style of lecture films from the Korean War and World War II, was in itself something of an impossible charge. "Realism" as reflected in *Girls* is limited to what appeared to be real about Vietnam from the American military perspective—that the country was a fantastic, indecipherable, and dangerous territory, and that careful management of this experience, like the management of venereal disease, was required in order to return home intact in body and spirit. Management of the Vietnam experience could not and did not proceed from a basis of disengagement, but rather from a more complex *formulation* of imagined interactive possibilities—a model based on sexual fantasy and consumerist desire. Soldiers were taught the rules of *cautious engagement*—a strategy designed to enable their limited and pleasurable participation in the place of psychic displacement representing an imaginary, feminized Vietnam. Yet they were not taught how to use condoms, how to treat Vietnamese women respectfully, or how to conceptualize their own devastating experiences in larger-scale critical terms.

Where the Girls Are embodies the complex cross-purposes of military health-education cinema. On the one hand, it attempts to serve as an educational experience, designed to inform the serviceman about the avoidance of sexually transmitted infection. On the other hand, the film appears unable to escape from its own context, manifesting a cinematic form that mimics the imagery and stereotypes of contemporaneous sexualized fantasy in regards to Southeast Asia. As such, *Girls* demonstrates the potential unwitting complicity of preventive health education in stigmatizing ethnic and cultural differences as sites of disease. It provides evidence of the ongoing difficulty of institutionalized sexual-health education and highlights the challenge of creating complex, nonstereotypical film productions capable of eliciting positive behavioral change.

NOTES

1. *Where the Girls Are—VD in Southeast Asia*, prod. Jerry Warner, dir. Richard R. Miller, writ. William Lundgren, Jerry Warner and Associates, 1969. Archival sources in moving image and production files of the United States Air Force Aerospace Audio-Visual Service (USAF-AAVS) and Central Foreign Policy Files of the General Records of the Department of State, held by the National Archives at College Park, MD (hereinafter cited as NA-CP).

2. Susan Jeffords, *The Remasculinization of America: Gender and the Vietnam War* (Bloomington: Indiana University Press, 1989), xi–xi.

3. Laura Mulvey, "Visual Pleasure and Narrative Cinema," *Screen* 16, no. 3 (1975): 6–18.

4. Catherine Hill, "Planning for Prostitution: An Analysis of Thailand's Sex Industry," in *Women's Lives and Public Policy: The International Experience*, ed. Meredeth Turshen and Briavel Holcomb (Westport, CT: Praeger, 1993), 134–5; and the *Washington Post*, October 23, 1969, enclosed in Memo to File; General Subject Files, 1960–9; Records of the Office of the Surgeon General (Army), Record Group 112; NA-CP. Brigadier General David T. Thomas, Surgeon General, Commander of the 44th Medical Brigade, suggests that the military should operate houses of prostitution in order to reduce venereal disease rates among soldiers. Thomas notes, "[elimination of prostitution] is a policy that reportedly is winked at by a number of commanders and medical officers in Vietnam."

5. Allan M. Brandt, *No Magic Bullet: A Social History of Venereal Disease in the United States Since 1880* (New York: Oxford University Press, 1985), 175–8.

6. Saundra Sturdevant and Brenda Stoltzfus, "Disparate Threads of the Whole: An Interpretative Essay," in *Let the Good Times Roll: Prostitution and the U.S. Military in Asia* (New York: New Press, 1992), 300–34, 305.

7. *Sex Hygiene*, dir. John Ford, prod. Darryl F. Zanuck, 1941. Held at NA-CP.

8. Report, Form DS 322, Narcotics: Heroin Usage by GI's in Vietnam, May 1973; General Records of the Department of State, Central Foreign Policy Files, 1967–9, Record Group 59, Folder Soc 11–5 VietS; NA-CP.

9. Brandt, 164; Thomas A. Verdon and Evan T. Thomas, "Current Problems with Neisseria Gonorrhea in Vietnam," *USARV Medical Bulletin*, USARV Pamphlet No. 40–22 (July–August 1970): 9; and *Preventive Medicine in Vietnam, 1965–1966: Proceedings of a Symposium of the Office of the Surgeon, United States Army, Vietnam*, ed. LTC Robert J. T. Joy, Chief, U.S.A. Medical Research Team (WRAIR) Vietnam, June 27–28, 1966, Records of the Office of the Surgeon General (Army), General Subject Files, 1960–9, Record Group 112, Box 106, Preventive Medicine Subject File; NA-CP.

10. Hal Albert, Acting DCS/Operations, Norton Air Force Base, California, to 1350th Motion Picture Squadron, Wright-Patterson Air Force Base, Ohio, July 10, 1968; Records of United States Air Force Commands, Activities, and Organization,

Record Group 342, Folder SFP 1867–84 (hereinafter after cited as USAF-AAVS); NA-CP; and Rolland V. Beech, Chief, Commercial Production Unit, 1350th Motion Picture Squadron, to Ray Ussery, Supervising Producer, Aerospace Audio-Visual Service, Norton Air Force Base, July 16, 1968, USAF-AAVS; NA-CP.

11. Cliff E. Raisor, Special Assistant for Information, Office of the Surgeon General, to Colonel James P. Warndorf, Vice Commander, Aerospace Audio-Visual Service, Norton Air Force Base, October 21, 1968, USAF-AAVS; NA-CP.

12. Col. Robert R. Burwell, Command Representative, United States Air Force, Washington DC, Draft Film Script with Motion Picture Production Request and Film Requirements, May 31, 1968, USAF-AAVS; NA-CP.

13. Commander in Chief, Pacific Air Force, telegram, November 22, 1968, USAF-AAVS; NA-CP.

14. Delivery of the first 250 advance release prints to Norton Air Force Base was accomplished on April 28, 1969.

15. Albert to 1350th Motion Picture Squadron, July 10, 1968. Beech to Ussery, July 16, 1968. Ray Ussery, Pre-Script/Treatment Conference Report, July 30, 1968, USAF-AAVS; NA-CP.

16. Video Yesteryear, in Sandy Hook, MA, and Traditions Military Videos, in San Diego, CA.

17. William E. Murdoch, Contracting/Ordering Officer, 1350th, to Milner-Fenwick, Inc., Baltimore, MD, Appendix A to Motion Picture Script Contract/Purchase Order F33660-68-A-0070, July 17, 1968, USAF-AAVS; NA-CP.

18. Jerry Warner, Executive Producer, Warner and Associates, Los Angeles, CA, to William E. Murdoch, Contracting Officer, Aerospace Audio-Visual Service, Norton Air Force Base, January 22, 1969, USAF-AAVS; NA-CP.

19. Trinh T. Minh-ha, *When the Moon Waxes Red* (New York: Routledge, 1991), 81–105.

20. Johannes Fabian, *Time and the Other: How Anthropology Makes Its Object* (New York: Columbia University Press, 1983), 6–7.

21. Neil L. Jamieson, *Understanding Vietnam* (Berkeley: University of California Press, 1993), 339.

22. *The Women Outside: Korean Women and the U.S. Military,* Orinne J. T. Takagi and Hye Jung Park/Third World Newsreel, 1995, 60 min. 16 mm. Third World Newsreel, New York, NY (aired on PBS television, July 16, 1996).

23. Thomas A. Bass, *Vietnamerica: The War Comes Home* (New York: Soho Press, 1996), 33.

24. Ibid.

25. American Embassy, Saigon, Saigon Night Life Faces an Evolution, December 21, 1967; General Records of the Department of State, Record Group 59, Subject-Numeric Files, Central Foreign Policy Files, 1967–9; NA-CP.

26. American Embassy, Saigon Night Life Faces an Evolution, December 21, 1967.

27. Ibid.

28. Caroline Dunn, *The Politics of Prostitution in Thailand and the Philippines: Policies and Practice,* Working Paper 86 (Clayton, Victoria, Australia: Centre of Southeast Asian Studies, Monash University, 1994), 13.

29. Jamieson, 352, 333.

30. Brandt, 101, 119.

31. Burwell, Draft Film Script with Motion Picture Production Request and Film Requirements, May 31, 1968.

32. American Embassy, Saigon Night Life Faces an Evolution, December 21, 1967.

33. For a discussion of how Vietnamese women were viewed as prostitutes, see Renny Christopher, *The Viet Nam War/The American War: Images and Representations in Euro-American and Vietnamese Exile Narratives* (Amherst: University of Massachusetts Press, 1995), 141.

34. Prostitution was illegal in Vietnam and three to four hundred girls were arrested by the Saigon police each day. These women were not checked for gonorrhea and syphilis prior to release. Street penicillin was available and complicated treatment by either instilling a false sense of having been treated or inducing the proliferation of resistant microorganisms. Military surveys in Vietnam in 1969 and 1970 indicated that 50–60 percent of bar girls at in-country R&R sites were infected with gonorrhea. In contrast to American soldiers who could report to a physician, women who had contracted resistant disease strains had no medical options, due to the Vietnamese government's lack of acknowledgement of the prostitution industry and its willingness to prosecute these women as criminals.

35. Ray Ussery, Record of Verbal Coordination with Lt. Col. Paul Nugent, Technical Advisor, U.S. Air Force, Washington DC, November 21, 1968, USAF-AAVS; NA-CP.

36. Ray Ussery, Memo for the Record, October 22, 1968, USAF-AAVS; NA-CP.

37. Terry Collins, "The Vietnam War, Reascendent Conservatism, White Victims," *Postmodern Culture* 2, no. 3 (1992), http://muse.jhu.edu/journals/postmodern_culture/v002/2.3r_collins.html (accessed November 29, 2003).

38. Burwell, Draft Film Script with Motion Picture Production Request and Film Requirements, May 31, 1968.

39. Thomas E. Farmer, Operations Assistant for the Commander, AVODOM, Production of SFP 1873, December 15, 1968, USAF-AAVS; NA-CP. Roland V. Beech to Ray Ussery, Production of SFP 1873 with attached Scene Description List, December 17, 1968, USAF-AAVS; NA-CP.

40. Ray Ussery, Pre-Script/Treatment Conference Report, July 30, 1968.

41. Thomas E. Farmer, Production of SFP 1873, December 15, 1968. Beech to Ussery, Production of SFP 1873 with attached Scene Description List, December 17, 1968.

42. Alton F. Grun, Executive Officer, 1352nd Photo Group, Lookout Mountain Air Force Station, Los Angeles, CA, to Ray Ussery, Norton Air Force Base, Information on Stock Footage, December 30, 1968, USAF-AAVS; NA-CP. Ray Ussery, Record of Coordination with Don Locks of Lookout Mountain Film Library, December 30, 1968, USAF-AAVS; NA-CP.

43. Burwell, Draft Film Script with Motion Picture Production Request and Film Requirements, May 31, 1968.

44. Linda Williams, *Hard Core: Power, Pleasure, and the "Frenzy of the Visible"* (Berkeley: University of California Press, 1989), 130–1.

45. Ibid., 134.

46. Brandt, 164.

47. Joseph Magro, Chief, Commercial Production Section, to Roland V. Beech, January 16, 1969, USAF-AAVS; NA-CP; and Jerry Warner, Executive Producer, Warner and Associates, Los Angeles, CA, to William E. Murdoch, Contracting Officer, Aerospace Audio-Visual Service, Norton Air Force Base, Summary: Contract Additions and Modifications; additional costs, February 6, 1969, USAF-AAVS; NA-CP.

48. The total budget for the finished film, including the cost of 16 mm release prints delivered to the Air Force, was $46,362.28. The overrun was approximately $12,000.

49. Brigadier General Wallace K. Wittwer, Provost Marshal, United States Army, to Col. Noel, Surgeon, United States Army - Vietnam, May 29, 1971; Records of the Office of the Surgeon General (Army), Record Group 112; NA-CP.

50. Allen J. Seeber, "Controlled Prostitution Tried in Some U.S. Units," *U.S. Medicine* 7, no. 9 (1971): 1.

51. Suzanne Poirier, *Chicago's War on Syphilis, 1937–1940: The Times, The Trib, and the Clap Doctor* (Urbana: University of Illinois Press, 1995), 209.

52. Brandt, 164–5.

53. Memo to File, Attachment to Performance Period Report - Rough Cut Phase, February 28, 1969, USAF-AAVS; NA-CP.

54. Burwell, Draft Film Script with Motion Picture Production Request and Film Requirements, May 31, 1968.

55. Ibid.

56. Ray Ussery, Memo for the Record, April 1, 1969, USAF-AAVS; NA-CP.

57. Ray Ussery, TDY Report on Production Planning Conference, December 11, 1968, USAF-AAVS; NA-CP.

58. John S. Wolf, Consular Officer, Danang, Foreign Service Office, Mixed-Blood Children in MR I, enclosed in Airgram, August 23, 1973; General Records of the Department of State, Record Group 59, Subject-Numeric Files, Central Foreign Policy Files, 1967–1969; NA-CP.

59. Ibid.

60. Cynthia Enloe, *Bananas, Beaches, and Bases: Making Feminist Sense of International Politics* (Berkeley: University of California Press, 1990), 35–6.

61. Ibid., 41.

Bug Chasing, Barebacking, and the Risks of Care

Gregory Tomso

barebacking (n.): intentional unprotected anal sex

bug chasing (n.): intentional unprotected anal sex performed in order to become infected with HIV

gift giving (n.): intentional unprotected anal sex performed in order to infect another person with HIV

Responding to what some experts and activists are calling a failure of public health, practitioners in the fields of public health, psychology, and sociology have recently turned their attention to the emerging phenomena of barebacking and bug chasing.[1] They are motivated by an altruism that aims to stop the spread of HIV and to protect the lives of those whose behaviors may expose them to the virus. Gay activists, too, are interested in these relatively new sexual behaviors. Some see them as proof of a proclivity toward self-destructive, sexual excess inherent to gay life while others regard barebacking and bug chasing as powerful acts of political resistance to conventional sexual morality and scientific orthodoxy.[2] Popular journalists have also turned their attention to these practices, using lurid graphics and fear-mongering prose to sensationalize them for mass-market audiences.[3] In short, barebacking and bug chasing have emerged as important catalysts in ongoing popular and professional debates over the meanings of gay sexuality and epidemic disease, and they offer a compelling point of entry for investigating the social and political dimensions of public health and social science.

This essay looks closely at contemporary accounts of bug chasing and barebacking across a wide range of venues, media, and genres. It begins with the assumption, drawn from critical science studies and discourse studies, that bug chasing and barebacking exist *as phenomena*

largely because of what Foucault would call the constitutive, disciplinary operation of scientific, activist, and popular discourses about them.[4]
This is to say that those who are currently investigating and writing
about these phenomena, as much so if not more than the men whose
sexual lives are the subjects of these investigations, are epistemologi-
cally accountable for the emergence of bug chasing and barebacking as
social "problems." A corollary to this assumption is that bug chasing
and barebacking are not manifestations of an empirical crisis to be
solved but, at the level of discourse itself, that they are terms whose
meanings and referents cannot be taken for granted. What, exactly,
makes bug chasing and barebacking so frightening and so powerful for
those who write about them? What can we learn about the formation
of sexual knowledge—and in particular about the construction of gay
identity—from these recent debates?

To answer these questions, I will compare accounts of bug chasing
and barebacking in mainstream magazines like *Poz* and *Rolling Stone*
with scientific articles from a variety of health-related fields. These
seemingly disparate sources all draw upon what might be called a
cultural unconscious of gay male sexuality. They employ common
rhetorical tropes, such as depicting the Internet as a breeding ground
for sexual deviance. They also rely on explicitly emotional and moral
modes of argumentation. In addition, both popular and scientific accounts provide evidence of a renewed social interest in investigating
and policing gay men's sexual "intentions," an interest that often
collapses the conceptual distinction between barebacking and bug chasing. Finally, these emerging discourses seem motivated, at least in part,
by a prurient interest in gay male sex that may be the result of cultural
anxieties about anal penetration and a growing fascination with gay sex
as an erotics of suicide and murder. As an article in *Rolling Stone*
recently put it, bug chasers are men "in search of death."[5]

In teasing out the overlapping strands of discourse surrounding
barebacking and bug chasing, we can see more clearly how these
phenomena both shape and are shaped by larger cultural understandings of gay sexuality. Of particular interest in this regard are signs, as
I will discuss in detail, of a seemingly irresolvable ethical dilemma that
emerges from the troubled intersection of public-health imperatives and
new modes of gay self-expression. This dilemma takes the form of a
double bind of care and violence in which caring for those at risk of
HIV infection can be seen as a violent limitation of gay men's freedom.
I mean freedom here not only at the level of individual choice or action
but also, philosophically speaking, at the level of gay ontology: the very
possibility of gay "being."

I. A Philosophy of the Question

What makes them do it? It seems impossible today to have a conversation about bug chasing or barebacking without hearing someone raise the question, "What makes them do it?"[6] While the tone of the question may change, the desire that motivates the question is generally the same. In scientific and popular literature alike, there is an ever-growing interest in uncovering and cataloging the reasons why men who "know better" continually engage in these taboo sexual behaviors. The list of reasons is already expansive: low self-esteem; the physical pleasures of condomless sex; a "culture of disease" created by glossy HIV-medication ads that equate infection with "popularity and acceptance"; childhood sexual abuse; drug use; rebellion against authority; "sexual self-control deficits"; and the eroticization of risk itself, to name just a few.[7] While health experts continue to define the dimensions of these emerging phenomena in professional journals, it has become fashionable in mainstream media to feature lengthy exposés on the sexual recalcitrance of men who have sex with men. The infamous *Rolling Stone* article of February 6, 2003, "In Search of Death," is just one of many mass-marketed stories that have capitalized on Americans' fascination with the seemingly lurid details of gay men's sexual lives. The *New York Times Magazine*, for example, recently featured a story on the "down low" subculture of urban black men who, though sexually active with other men, view condoms as part of an effeminate, white gay culture that is at odds with traditional black masculinity.[8]

Whether focused at the level of biology, psychology, society, or culture, accounts of barebacking and bug chasing share a common structure and a common limit. As expressions of the desire to know "what makes them do it," these accounts always imagine the phenomena they describe as problems that need to be solved or as mysteries of human behavior that need to be understood and treated. This desire cannot be disentangled—indeed cannot be distinguished—from any empiricism or altruism that motivates inquiries into these mysteries. The question marks the entry of science and morality into the field of everyday lives, the lives of the men whose sexual and psychological habits have elicited curiosity, concern, fear, and rage in the minds of those who ask it. Not surprisingly, the tone of recent accounts is almost always one of crisis. In the case of the scientific literature, articles frequently include an urgent call for more research into the causes of intentional unprotected sex. More and better knowledge, it seems, will carry the day against the ravages of desire. In the popular press, the outcries are even louder, ranging from outright moral condemnation to fear mongering to compassionate yet righteous appeals to gay men to practice rationality and restraint.

Yet what would it mean to suspend the question that structures these accounts? By refusing to answer the question, we can open an inquiry into the nature of the question itself, asking how it functions simultaneously as an instrument of science, an expression of desire, a rhetorical trope, and, metaphysically speaking, an act of violence toward gay men. Such a refusal allows, in short, for what might be called a theory of the question. This is also a theory of the violence of desire itself: not, that is, the violence of gay desire, but the violence that belongs to wanting to know something about another, the Other, who is not the self.[9]

Yet the question "What makes them do it?" is also the opening of ethics, defined here as the possibility of care for the Other. Without the question, there is no means for reflection, no grounds for action, no possibility for prevention. In an era of crisis and devastating loss, the question conveys, among other sentiments, the feeling that something must be done. But what is the relationship between this care, this ethics, and the violence that the question entails? Is it possible, in the midst of this particular epidemic, to separate care from violence?

In his essay "Violence and Metaphysics," Jacques Derrida offers a meditation on the relationship between ethics and violence that helps to answer these questions. He writes of philosophy's "unbreachable responsibility" to pose questions in such a way that "the hypocrisy of an answer" is not yet "fraudulently articulated within the very syntax of the question" (80). This call for a philosophy of ethical responsibility, of what Derrida also calls "nonviolence," is useful in thinking through the vexing and highly politicized questions of identity and language that shape the discourses of bug chasing and barebacking. At the center of his investigations, Derrida places the problem of the relationship between self and Other. He asks if it is possible to see or even to conceive of the Other without in some way diminishing the Other's freedom. He describes ethics as the "permitting to *let* be others in their truth" (146, Derrida's italics). This letting be of others is "as close as possible to nonviolence" as one can ever come: "*We do not say pure nonviolence*. Like pure violence, pure nonviolence is a contradictory concept" (146, Derrida's italics).[10] If we wish to preserve our own dignity as well as the dignity of the Other, if we wish to meet our ethical responsibility toward the Other, we must, Derrida suggests, commit violence against the Other. The path of nonviolence is opened by violence itself.

To the extent that it structures current accounts of bug chasing and barebacking, the question "What makes them do it?" is the opposite of letting be. What is to be revealed by the question brings to mind what Andrew Sullivan has referred to as the "deep and dark psychological reasons" of those who wish to infect themselves with HIV.[11] Yet if we temper the desire to see inside these seemingly troubled minds and the sordid subcultures that supposedly nurture them, we might note something of the structure of the fetish in our relationship to them: a cathexis of thought and energy invested not in fully differentiated Others but formed around a dark and threatening mass that, as if a thing unto itself, is what we call "gay desire." We might also pose a second question, a question for metaphysics, that concerns the possibility of the opening of thought around gay desire. That question might look something like this: Can we speak of bug chasing and barebacking *at all* without perpetuating some form of homophobic violence? The answer is simple: there is no nonviolent articulation, nor can there be, of bug chasing or barebacking as such. Yet this "no" is not the endpoint of ethical inquiry. It is a recognition of the violence toward the Other that, in the Derridean sense, is the beginning of the ethical relationship as such. It is within the constraints of this violent beginning that the language of science and of popular reporting assumes its importance and becomes worthy of our attention.

II. The Discourses of Barebacking and Bug Chasing

One of the benefits of discourse analysis, a popular methodology in the emerging field of cultural studies, is that it allows researchers to identify the "shared assumptions that function to make discourse comprehensible and meaningful."[12] Such analysis highlights the ideological, structural (grammatical and syntactical), cultural, and psychological moorings of language. It often brings to bear on nonfiction texts, such as scientific reports or news accounts, the tools of literary analysis. By looking for similarities in a range of texts from a variety of different contexts, discourse analysis provides a "big picture" view of how meaning is created, shared, and transformed.

One of the most striking aspects of contemporary discourse about bug chasing and barebacking is the absence of what might have been an important distinction between the two.[13] The elision of barebacking, or any act of unprotected intercourse, into what is generally portrayed as the morally repugnant and antisocial practice of bug chasing, in which gay men wantonly (or so the story goes) seek their own deaths, is made possible in part because of a refusal to take seriously the facts that, first, unprotected receptive anal intercourse between men does not inevitably lead to HIV infection and, second, that unprotected intercourse is most often a heterosexual phenomenon. (Among men who have sex with men in the United States, the probability of being infected with HIV during unprotected, receptive anal intercourse with an HIV-positive partner has been estimated to be anywhere from .5 percent to 30 percent depending on what phase of HIV infection is present in the already positive partner.[14]) Mark Blechner writes:

> [The term barebacking] comes from the equestrian world, where riding bareback is wild, dangerous, and fun. In the sexual world, when you think of barebacking, do you think of your mother and father having intercourse? Probably not. The implication of barebacking, at least in the United States, is that it is unprotected anal intercourse between gay men, in a context in which there is some danger of HIV-infection.[15]

Barebacking has come to be equated with the gay male anus and involves a particular kind of desire that is wild, dangerous, and reckless. It is hardly possible today to speak of barebacking without the implicit or explicit feeling that, in both the act and the very imagination of the act, a wrong is being committed.

Some public-health researchers and psychologists have taken care to construct more rigorous definitions of barebacking, most often focusing on the presence or absence of subjective intent: "A key aspect of this definition is intent: the individual consciously seeks unprotected anal sex."[16] Such formal discriminations between intentionally having unprotected anal sex (barebacking) and intentionally having unprotected anal sex *in order to place the self or someone else at risk of infection* (bug chasing) are not, however, as conceptually distinct as one might wish. The move to define barebacking strictly as intentional unsafe sex can only be achieved by bringing barebacking conceptually closer to bug chasing, making barebacking a psychological concern that requires assessment and intervention as a problem of volition or desire. My own use of the terms barebacking and bug chasing in tandem throughout this essay is meant to mark their collapse into one another and to suggest that anxieties around both phenomena share a common cultural origin in fears of gay men's "intentions" toward others as well as in fears of the anus as a site of death.[17]

To speak, then, of bug chasing and barebacking is to speak exclusively not only of gay male desire but of gay male desire of a very dangerous kind. One of the earliest and most striking representations of such desire appeared in the February 1999 issue of *POZ* magazine, a periodical marketed to people living with HIV and AIDS. The issue included two stories on barebacking, each framed by a series of provocative graphics depicting barebackers, quite literally, as sexual and moral cowboys.[18] One image, for example, shows Tony Valenzuela, "the first openly HIV positive porn actor in the United States," standing naked, outdoors, alongside a saddleless horse (50). The "rawness" and naturalness of Valenzuela's unclothed body connects him to the wildness of the horse and the forest path down which it walks. Both studs, the image implies, are happiest and most virile when they are not "saddled" by leather or latex.

"They Shoot Barebackers, Don't They?," the title of the story this image accompanies, is a titillating play on the title of Horace McCoy's 1935 novel, *They Shoot Horses, Don't They?* Ironically and angrily, this title asks readers to imagine barebackers' deaths not from AIDS-related illnesses, but, presumably, from the readers' own murderous desires to shoot barebackers for their (equally murderous) sins of sexual recklessness. The implicit reference to McCoy's novel intensifies this suggestion of murder, since the novel tells the story of a man named Robert who is about to be sentenced for the death of a woman named Gloria, but the connections do not end here:

> We discover that the murder Robert is sentenced for isn't really a murder, since it was Gloria who, after 36 consecutive and nightmarish days and nights, asked him to kill her and gave him the gun for him to do so. In fact it's a "helped" suicide, some kind of violent euthanasia. But Robert did it with no witness around him. He did it because it seemed natural to him, with the memory of a horse shot the same way by his grandfather when he was a kid. At a moment, during his trial, he remembers and feels sorry and stupid about his foolish and fatal act.[19]

Similarly, the logic of barebacking implicit in this issue of *POZ* reads as follows: barebackers kill because "it seems natural to them"; they are assisting one another in "some kind of violent euthanasia" or "suicide"; and when called to account for their actions, they will feel "sorry and stupid" for their "foolish and fatal" acts. While neither of the two articles nor the editorial that accompanies them actually goes this far in its moral questioning of barebacking, the issue's graphics, along with the articles' titles, perform the work of tacit moral condemnation.

This condemnation seems, in many instances, at odds with the magazine's ostensibly progressive stance towards barebacking, evidenced by a list of "Safer Barebacking Considerations" authored by the "HIV-negative prevention activist" Michael Scarce. Scarce, whose story "A Ride on the Wild Side" is the second feature article, nominally maintains the distinction between barebacking and bug chasing. Yet whatever steps Scarce takes to separate the two are undone by the article's lurid title as well as by its primary graphic, a giant red circle and slash over the word "rubbers," both of which, once again, create a link between barebacking and wild, morally reckless behavior (figure 1).

The graphic furthers this link for readers through its inclusion of a small dotted line that runs down the bound side of the page on which it is printed, suggesting that the entire page might be cut out and displayed. In an ironic reversal of its own moralizing headlines, the magazine seemingly promotes barebacking even as it sets out to sensationalize it. The decision not to use condoms becomes, in this instance, a literal badge of pride and accomplishment.

The article itself, written in the first person, tells the story of Scarce's research trip to a barebacking party in the Castro district of San Francisco. At times both thoughtful and nonmoralizing—"[t]hese experiences have led me to believe that barebackers do not deserve to be vilified, but rather more fully understood"(71)—Scarce's claims to objectivism are undercut by the story's edgy graphics and, as it turns out, by Scarce's very presence in the role of first-person narrator. The fact that he is HIV negative, for example, is advertised in large print just above the article's title, suggesting that this status qualifies him to investigate the issues at hand, as if someone who is HIV positive could not be as objective as someone who is uninfected. Yet readers soon learn that Scarce gives in to "temptation" during the barebacking party, but only by doing "what I usually do in the absence of condoms—blowjobs" (71). He then goes on to write of his own "intense emotions" during and after the party: "fascination, desire and dread" (71). These emotions reach their peak when he finally mentions bug chasers, calling them "[r]are exceptions to the barebacking norm" and congratulating himself on pressing one forty-five-year-old gift giver named Paul to confess the "twisted romantic nature" of his relationship with a twenty-one-year-old bug chaser (70). In his final word on the subject, Scarce confesses that Paul's "tone of voice, so matter-of-fact, is almost as disturbing to me as what he has to say" (70). This "disturbing" moment

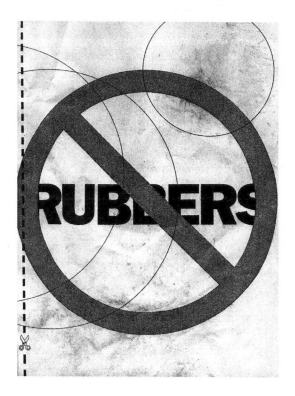

Figure 1. Graphic by Brian Carden. From *Poz*, February 1999. Reprinted with permission. Copyright 1999 Smart+Strong L.L.C.

of personal truth telling leaves bug chasing not, as Scarce might hope, having been thoughtfully or objectively analyzed but instead shrouded in mystery, nonunderstanding, and disbelief. Scarce's writing takes on the air of a Christian mystery story, a passion of temptation, sin, and imperfect redemption in which the moral transformation of the writer's self becomes the narrative's most important subject.

Though not a formal, scientific study of barebacking or bug chasing, Scarce's article draws from his interest in and commitment to public-health initiatives within various gay communities. While it would be unreasonable to read the article as representative of the state of the social and health sciences in relation to barebacking and bug chasing, it does seem reasonable to suggest that it points to a shared character-istic of nearly all writing about these phenomena, both popular and scientific: namely, that such writing sometimes sacrifices objectivity or moral neutrality in favor of what in literary parlance might be called sentiment. Such is the case in one scientific study published in the *Journal of the Association of Nurses in AIDS Care*:

> Many barebackers report a desire to either stay HIV negative or to protect partners from infection. What is more frightening is the reportedly small group of men actively seeking to become HIV infected ("bug chasers") or to infect others ("gift givers"). Scarce (1999) reported about the Web site "XtremeSex," which caters to this group of men and highlights the purported erotic appeal of HIV-infected semen. In addition, "XtremeSex" sex provides a forum for hundreds of personal ads for men seeking to become infected or to infect others.[20]

Like Scarce, whose *Poz* article is the report mentioned in this excerpt, the authors of this study betray their own emotional response to both barebacking and bug chasing: if barebacking is scary, bug chasing, as they put it, is even "more frightening." Moments like this one draw attention to the role of the self and its fears and desires in motivating and shaping the work of science. Is it possible, we might ask, to act out of altruism and out of fear at the same time? If not, then what constitutes the public good, and ultimately the public's health, is a matter sometimes decided by the private experience of sentiment rather than a collective one of rational decision making.

In its citing of Scarce's article from *Poz*, the study excerpted above also points to the way in which the distinctions between scientific and popular discourses can become blurred. Scientific writing about these phenomena frequently cite nonscientific essays as credible sources of information, in large part because popular or lay writers are seen to possess the most up-to-date information about gay culture.[21] As one team of researchers noted, scientific reporting might include anecdotes from popular media in order to "humanize" scientific research. In his book *Impure Science*, Steven Epstein demonstrates how scientific knowledge is the product of political negotiations among a variety of actors, including scientists from a variety of fields and lay "experts" who learn the language of science in order to challenge its assumptions, methods, and outcomes.[22] He emphasizes the intensely social, we might say the intensely human, processes by which scientific ideas and methods gain or lose their credibility. Looking at AIDS research from the perspective of discourse analysis, we can see yet another way in which scientific knowledge is formed through a series of interactions with that which is thought to be "external" to science. To "humanize" science by making reference to popular gay writers not only acknowledges the political pressures that activists have placed on scientists but also, at the level of writing itself, explicitly marks the hybridity of discourses that, above and beyond the role of any particular actor or group of actors, further blurs the distinction between expert and lay forms of knowledge. Such hybridity is not detrimental to the work of science; rather, it is an indication that science needs to be understood *as discourse.* "Science" is an aggregate of ways of speaking, thinking, and writing that shares the tropes and conventions of all other discourses.

One common trope that ties together much scientific and popular writing on barebacking and bug chasing is the portrayal of the Internet as a catalyst and breeding ground for dangerous sexual desires and practices. Researchers cite the recent emergence of Web sites such as XtremeSex.com, mentioned above, Barebacksex.com, Barebackcity.com, and Bareback.com (to name just a few) as an indication of how popular these practices are becoming. DeAnn K. Gauthier and Craig J. Forsyth have argued "that sometimes advances in technology may lead to unsafe sex. Thus, computer access to the Internet may encourage discussions of virtual sex (whether these discussions concern voyeurism, pedophilia, or bug chasing), which may in turn lead to dangerous, exploitative, or even unsafe real sex."[23] The authors add that the Internet facilitates such "behavioral exchanges," almost suggesting that it could transmit the bodily fluids, if not also the virus, supposedly sought by barebackers and bug chasers. Even more suggestive, and equally mystifying, is the parenthetical reference to "voyeurism, pedophilia, or bug chasing" as comparable forms of sexual deviance "encouraged" by access to the Internet. The implication here is not only that computers themselves might goad people into action but that bug chasing is a "dangerous, exploitative" behavior on a par with child molestation. Finally, the dichotomy created here between "discussions of virtual sex" and "real sex" (whatever that might be) is dubious, suggesting that the Internet is a breeding ground for high rates of deviance that otherwise might not exist in "real" life. This study not only reproduces conventional sexphobic and homophobic assumptions about the role of the Internet in fostering sexual perversity and promiscuity but also voices an anxiety about sexual discourse itself, as if discussing sex, virtually or otherwise, already assumes a certain amount of risk.

A more recent example of how the Internet functions as a trope in discussions of barebacking and bug chasing can be found in the

February 6, 2003, issue of *Rolling Stone* magazine. *Rolling Stone*'s now infamous feature-length story "In Search of Death" titillated readers with the alarming—and as it turns out fabricated—claim that "at least 25 percent of all newly infected gay men" consciously or subconsciously seek the virus that causes AIDS (48).[24] The story's leading graphic is a hazy image of a presumably gay, Latino man in his late twenties or early thirties sitting naked on a large bed, legs spread, his laptop computer placed squarely and comfortably across his genitals. The screen of the laptop displays a series of mathematical symbols, a field of small minus signs flowing gently into a field of small plus signs, meant here, it seems, to signify the desired transformation in his serostatus from HIV negative to HIV positive. The symbols might also signify the threat that the Internet presents to the HIV-negative world since it is through online chat rooms and barebacking Web sites that bug chasers and their positive counterparts, gift givers, frequently find one another. The virus itself seems to leak out of the computer screen, filling the air with a kind of infectious ether.

A morally censorious and fear-mongering tone is struck not only in the article's title but also in the sidebars that accompany the article and in the full-page advertisement that immediately follows it. One sidebar, bearing the caption "There's no Magic Pill," features a hand holding a small mountain of pills that are described as a "daily medication load" for someone living with "advanced" HIV (47). Each pill has a corresponding description, giving precisely two pieces of information about it: the name of the drug and its known side effects. Nothing is said about the power of these drugs to fight the progress of HIV or how thousands of people with HIV who take these drugs are living healthier lives even though HIV infection itself remains incurable. The omission of these and other details makes this "informational" sidebar seem less like objective fact reporting and more like a hit-and-run "we know better campaign" meant to refute the supposedly common assumption by bug chasers that HIV is now a chronic, manageable disease. "[D]espite some chasers' opinions," the sidebar reads, "HIV is a brutal and deadly disease. . . . [W]hen a carrier isn't struggling with the virus' symptoms . . . a life on meds involves a mind-numbing routine" (47). The sidebar's reference to those infected with HIV as "carriers" plays on the idea that people with HIV are malevolent beings, lurking on the Internet and elsewhere, waiting for their chance to infect the innocent. Another sidebar, entitled "Assault with a deadly Virus," metaphorically suggests that HIV is the deadly *weapon* that these HIV perpetrators will use to inflict harm on their unsuspecting victims (48).

On the page facing immediately opposite the last page of the bug chasing article, the magazine's editors chose to print a full-page advertisement titled "Hot Spot: The Inside Story on Healthy Sex" (49). The placement of this ad, with its image of a white heterosexual couple captured in the act of love making, hardly seems coincidental. Its representation of romantic, sensual, and practically airbrushed heterosexuality and its promise of delivering the "inside story on healthy sex" become an immediate foil to the feature on bug chasing, which can now be read implicitly as the "inside story" on *unhealthy* (that is, homosexual) sex. In addition to this sexual corrective, the ad suggests a racial corrective as well, in its shift from the faceless Latino man depicted in the bug chasing article to the facial close-up of the white models. The picture of the white couple embraced in love making also emphasizes the isolation of the men pictured in the bug chasing article (in addition to the Latino man, there is a portrait of a young white man) who, presented only in solo portraits, seem to embody the very antisociality of their desires. The overall effect of the February 6 issue, in its content, layout, and advertising—not to mention its release just prior to Valentine's Day—is of a crying out against the seeming insanity of gay male sex in the morally correct voice of normative heterosexuality.

Given these discursive effects, one might be more understanding of the Rev. Louis P. Sheldon, chairman of the Traditional Values Coalition, when he writes in his response to the *Rolling Stone* article that both barebackers and bug chasers "are apparently actively seeking death and are also willing to kill others as part of a sickening 'erotic' thrill."[25] Sheldon makes this statement even after acknowledging that Dr. Bob Cabaj, the San Francisco public-health expert quoted in the *Rolling Stone* article, publicly denied the claim attributed to him in the article that linked 25 percent of new infection rates among gay men to bug chasing. For Sheldon, and for many others, the statistical facts of the matter are not, and never have been, the issue. His response to the *Rolling Stone* story bears a striking resemblance to the responses of two other national commentators on gay issues, Andrew Sullivan and Dan Savage. In a January 24 editorial on Salon.com, Sullivan calls bug chasing "a bizarre sub-cultural phenomenon" perpetrated by "clearly disturbed" individuals for "all sorts of deep and dark psychological reasons."[26] Savage, whose popular syndicated sex-advice column "Savage Love" appears regularly in a host of media outlets such as the *Village Voice* and Gay.com, pulls no punches in his outright condemnation of bug chasers and of recent public-health initiatives that seek to understand and speak to gay men's changing relationships to traditional "safe sex" messages:

[T]he education strategy in vogue at GMHC [Gay Men's Health Crisis] and other AIDS organizations is this: We must respect the decisions gay men make—up to and including the decision to get infected with HIV. . . . That strategy seems as bizarre as it does ineffective. Perhaps it's time for GMHC and other AIDS groups to start telling gay men the truth. Taking stupid sexual risks—even if risk turns you on—is reckless; anal sex on the first date—even with condoms—is a bad idea; giving someone HIV—even if he wants it— is immoral; being a huge . . . slut—as popular as that might make you—has physical and emotional consequences.[27]

What Savage appears to be indignant about here is the ever-growing acknowledgement in the fields of public health, sociology, and psychology that the "use a condom every time message" of 1980s safe-sex campaigns is not entirely effective and indeed has been subject to a powerful backlash in some gay male communities.[28] The looming failure of this public-health dogma led, in 2002, to the publication of *Beyond Condoms : Alternative Approaches to HIV Prevention*, edited by Ann O'Leary of the Centers for Disease Control and Prevention and intro-duced by Thomas Coates, director of the AIDS Research Institute at the University of California, San Francisco.[29] "[C]onsistent condom use," O'Leary writes in her preface to the volume, "is difficult for many individuals to achieve, and the prospect of a lifetime of this regimen is daunting to most of us."[30] While O'Leary's words may at this point be common knowledge among certain activists, public-health researchers, and care providers, there is a noticeable and contentious gap between this knowledge and the views of popular writers such as Savage, Sullivan, and Sheldon, who continue to pathologize and demonize the behaviors of those who have unprotected sex.

The larger point I would like to make here is not, however, about the disparities between expert and popular forms of knowledge but about the rhetorical similarities that tie together nearly all forms of discourse about barebacking and bug chasing: what literary critics would call the intertextuality of discourses that draw on a shared body of rhetorical tropes, such as the association of gay sex and death. The power of this trope is that it is not limited to the sensationalism of the popular press; rather, it functions to advance the arguments of scientific writing as well. Consider the following claim from a study in the journal *Deviant Behavior*: "The HIV-negative individuals sometimes feel such isolation as a result [of not being infected] that they wish to become members of their community again, regardless of the cost. They are willing to commit what is, in essence, suicide in order to maintain their membership in the group."[31] While it is undeniable that many gay men experience intense feelings of guilt and shame—even suicidal ones—the dubiousness of this study's rhetoric lies in its failure to separate discussion of these feelings from discussion of potentially unsafe sexual acts. Thus, the authors achieve a rather remarkable sleight of hand in the placement of the phrase "in essence," which magically equates unsafe sexual acts with intentionally suicidal ones. While the meanings of all acts that we consider to be sexual are rooted in personal and social contexts, including those of shame, the authors here singularly reduce the meaning of sex to seeking death.

The discourses of barebacking and bug chasing suggest that the link between gay male sex and death is as strong today as ever. Its perseverance is hardly surprising since it comes as a murderous extension of the bourgeois medicalization in the eighteenth and nineteenth centuries of homosexuality and other perversions, such as masturbation, as wasteful forms of nonreproductive sexuality.[32] Whereas death was once viewed only as a possible and extreme outcome of the moral and physical debility that resulted from wasteful sexual spending, barebacking and bug chasing, in a new, almost elegantly simplistic twist on this centuries-old theme, now make death the inevitable endpoint of male-male sexuality while formally inscribing a desire for death and murder at the very heart of contemporary gay identity. If we take Freud's theory of the death drive seriously, and acknowledge a general desire for death underlying all of human behavior, there is still reason to be suspicious of the particular linking of barebacking and bug chasing with a desire for death. Acknowledging a general human tendency toward self-destruction is not the same as endorsing the homophobic, rhetorical linkage of particular sexual acts (unprotected anal sex) by particular people (gay men) with a desire for particular acts of death (suicide and murder).

Even within the domain of what we might call expert or scientific knowledge there are significant uncertainties and disagreements about what desires, behaviors, individuals, and risks are meant to be signified by the terms barebacking and bug chasing. This uncertainty can be seen in an exchange in the *Journal of Gay and Lesbian Psychotherapy* in which Donna M. Orange and Mark J. Blechner, two experts in the field, respond to an article by J. P. Cheuvront about HIV-negative men who engage in high-risk sexual behaviors.[33] Based on the experience of his own psychotherapy practice, Cheuvront notes that "few patients who identify themselves as barebackers, or are in some other way committed to not taking steps to protect themselves from HIV infection, are HIV-negative" (19). He also writes that "my sense is that most risk-taking patients feel significant shame surrounding sexual risks they have taken," adding that "[r]isk taking is seldom, if ever, a planned behavior" (20). In his response, Blechner notes that he is "surprised by Cheuvront's assertion that, in his own practice, most people who engage in unsafe behavior are already HIV-positive" (30). "I am not sure," Blechner writes, "that we can generalize to the population at large" (30). He also expresses some doubt about Cheuvront's claim that most patients feel shame about taking sexual risks: "I cannot argue with the statistics of his [Cheuvront's] own practice, but I think that there are certainly many barebackers who are not ashamed of the sexual risks they have taken. On the contrary, they are proud and defiant, in what some see as courageous behavior against sexual repression and punitive attitudes, sometimes tinged with homophobia" (29). Meanwhile, Orange, in her reply to Cheuvront, takes issue with his claim that risk taking is seldom "a planned behavior": "[p]robably the conceptual problem here is that risk-taking is not a 'behavior' at all, but a property of a relational system" (48). On the one hand, if Cheuvront *is* correct about risk taking "seldom, if ever" being a planned behavior, then recent attempts in public-health science to define barebacking strictly as *intentional* unsafe intercourse are unlikely to help the majority of barebackers. On the other hand, if we take Orange's perspective, we see the difficulty of even defining the term "behavior" since it implies a certain agency or subjectivity that supposedly exists sui generis rather than as part of an interpersonal context or "relational system." Yet even Orange herself makes a rather sudden rhetorical leap in her response from discussing "the willingness of some gay men to take sexual risks" in one sentence to mentioning "this willingness-to-die and willingness-to-risk-the-death-of-others" in the next (46).

Even if these particular semantic and taxonomic difficulties could be settled, we would still be left with significant disagreements about the particular affects—shame, pride, defiance—that characterize sexual risk takers. What, ultimately, do the signifiers "bug chasing" and "barebacking" signify? Do they signify behaviors? Intentions? Psychologies? Emotions? Subcultures? Systems? The location of the signified in this semiotic system is unstable and indeed ever changing. Given the ethical and ontological stakes of these discourses, it might make sense to sort more rigorously through this messiness of signification before deciding which particular public-health strategies and care approaches will be most useful.

III. Queer Ethics

Part of the ethical difficulty embodied in the phenomena of barebacking and bug chasing is that, for many gay men, unprotected and risky sex are frequently life-affirming practices. Writers such as Eric Rofes, Michael Scarce, Michael Warner, Walt Odets, Mark Davis, J. P. Cheuvront, and others have attempted to describe the psychological, phenomenological, and sociological textures of gay men's lives in ways that position bug chasing and barebacking less as markers of pathological identity and more as behaviors motivated by ever-changing combinations of choices, blockages, fears, and desires that constitute both the life-affirming and life-denying practices of contemporary gay male life. These outlaw perspectives on unsafe sex provide, in the words of Scarce, "a more complex system of language with which to talk about sexuality and risk behavior."[34] As Rofes has noted, "Those who are having sex without condoms are not lacking in self-esteem or filled with internalized homophobia that triggers them to self-destruct."[35] Davis, a public-health researcher working with gay men in London, has written in the conclusion to his recent study of gay men's risk narratives that "lived risk is a productive complex of rationality, knowledge and meaning" in which more than one kind of rationality may be operative.[36] Cheuvront has argued that taking sexual risks can be an important part of "self-care." In each of these arguments, as in my own, there is a certain gay positivism at work, a witnessing of the trials and struggles of gay men to find place and identity through sex. These acts of witnessing presuppose something called "gayness" or, at the very least, something worth fighting for on behalf of all gay men. This positivism is a sign of the politicization of bug chasing and barebacking discourses. At stake is not only the health of gay men, but their very *survival*, a survival that exceeds the medical sense of the body's living or dying and entails the more symbolic, metaphysical sense of belonging to the describable and representable world. Derrida once asked if it were possible to feign speaking a language (89). In a related sense, we might ask how it is possible to care for an "at risk" population whose most powerful unity is ultimately an illusion of discourse.

My own aims in analyzing the discourses of bug chasing and barebacking are paradoxical. In attempting to stave off a certain violence toward gay men that seems inherent to contemporary discourse, I reify the very ontology of gayness over which I have cast a net of suspicion and scrutiny. I cannot resolve this paradox, and I see it as yet another instance of the Derridean double bind of care and violence discussed above. More generally, this paradox is only one of the many ways in which discourses of barebacking and bug chasing point to a larger problem or difficulty in queer ethics, one in which advocates for gay rights from a variety of different backgrounds and with a host of divergent and often conflicting professional and personal investments become polarized around debates about the status, meaning, and impact of unprotected sex. Underneath these debates is the larger, unanswerable question of gay identity itself.

The value of theory for me—and here I include discourse analysis as falling generally under the heading of theory—lies precisely in its potential to engage questions of ethics and even of politics without having to claim those questions in the terms in which they have been popularly or traditionally phrased. In this light, we might speak of the temporal as opposed to the objective dimensions of theory; that is, of theory as *chronos*, or the occasion for deliberation or doubt, rather than as *telos*, the definite outcome of any particular line of thought, investigation, program, policy, or action. Theory *makes* time by helping to show how the "question" of bug chasing and barebacking will never be fully answered, indeed that it cannot be, whether its answer lies in the call for more research, better communication, "urgently needed dialogue," more compassionate psychotherapy, community education, or the embracing of risky sex as a foundation for gay liberation or identity.[37] One senses here the old antagonism between "theory" and "practice." Theory *insists* on time, and this insistence is a key component of its ethics. Theory and practice thus represent two different ethics, one that is for time and one which is against. One *waits* while the other *does*. The very structure of this binary between waiting and doing is itself an ethical problem that cannot be resolved. In analyzing discourse, we become aware that what Derrida calls the "irreducible" divide between theory and praxis is not an end to, but the very instantiation of, ethical responsibility as the failed possibility of a nonviolent relation to the Other.[38]

One choice that such analysis opens before us is the possibility of distinguishing between the ethics and morality of discourse. The discourses I have examined here are ethical in that they are directed toward the care of the Other. They are also moral in that they prescribe various relationships to the Other that are, in the first instance, self-serving. There is value, I would argue, in making this distinction, first, because moral positions are not uncommon in both popular and scientific accounts of barebacking and bug chasing and, second, because doing so is one effective way of thinking more deeply about the ethical distinction between self and Other. Moral references in the popular media, from writers like Sheldon, Sullivan, and Savage, are obvious enough, yet the case is really no different in the scientific literature. For instance, Marshall Forstein, assistant professor of psychiatry at Harvard Medical School and chair of the Commission on AIDS of the American Psychiatric Association, makes the following distinction between high-risk behaviors in HIV-negative and HIV-positive men: "Although the meaning of the risky sexual behavior may be rooted in similar psycho-logical and social constructs for both the HIV negative and positive man who barebacks, the moral question remains, I believe, fundamentally different: it is one thing to decide to place oneself at risk, and quite another to do so to another person."[39] In a similar vein, Mark Blechner asks whether clinicians should "attend only to those individuals who experience conflict [because of their risky behaviors] and therefore seek psychotherapy? Or should we attend to the social phenomena that are endangering future generations?" (29) He goes on to answer his own question, admitting that "I don't think we as psychotherapists can ignore the social, and we may consider inserting our views into the debate about social norms" (32). For Blechner, this insertion means, in part, advocating for what amounts to be normative monogamous relationships for young gay men, who have, in his view, little contact with "long-term committed gay couples" who might serve as role models: "It seems a great loss to the gay community that there is not much more of a structure in place in which such couples can share their experiences and examples with younger men" (32). Forstein, who also writes in a more personal voice at the conclusion of his response, suggests:

> Each time a man makes love to another man, either as a detached body part of raw unbridled lust driven by the imperative of our sexual desire, or as the quest to merge self into other with the collective unconsciousness of the inevitable loneliness that is ulti-mately his alone to bear, he becomes the adventuring boy in search of his manhood, and in search of love. As therapists, we have a sacred responsibility to help each gay man feel entitled to his search for self and love, hoping to acknowledge the need for some risks while finding ways to diminish the danger, now symbolized by a retrovirus, that may foreshorten the journey to which each gay man is born. (42)

Forstein's language is sentimental ("the adventuring boy," "manhood," "inevitable loneliness"), mystical ("sacred," "journey," "quest"), and

highly prescriptive ("sacred responsibility"), qualities not normally associated with the discourses of science.

Alongside these writers' enlightened and compassionate responses
to bug chasing and barebacking, then, there is a distinct moral cen-
tralization or normalization that ultimately stands at odds with the
clinical positions they espouse. In Forstein's case in particular, the epic
tone of his conclusion and the poetic quality of his prose suggest an
attempt, through the very rhetoric and language of the essay itself, to
hold on to *or perhaps even to create* a kind of gay love that is both sacred
and endangered. As it draws deeply from spiritual and moral sources,
the language of science here enters what Judith Butler would call the
realm of the performative: language that, through an ongoing process
of citation and reiteration, calls into being that which it names or
describes.[40] Indeed, based on the articles examined here, we might say
that these sources performatively construct bug chasing and barebacking
as *moral* phenomena, since it is through the prescriptions and proscriptions of normative morality that these phenomena are named, referenced, and debated. They do not exist prior to this performative
construction but only through it, taking its name as their own.

Since the discourses of barebacking and bug chasing are only just
emerging and will undoubtedly proliferate in years to come, discourse
analysis will be one useful tool for thinking about their sometimes
conflicting ethical and moral dimensions. In earlier years of the AIDS
epidemic, those who studied scientific discourses urgently and rightly
called them to account for their racial, national, sexual, and gendered
biases.[41] As the social and cultural moorings of science become more
widely accepted, we might concentrate less on the politics of exposure
than on a consideration of ethics: on a consideration of how one might
best speak of and to the Other when all acts of speech seem destined
to end in violence, and yet when speech is essential for care and for
survival.[42] What makes sense, then, in the contexts of popular and
scientific writing is to build a movement toward a more responsible
discourse, a more responsible question. This responsibility does not
necessarily entail demanding a more rigorous adherence to truth or fact;
the patent falsity of *Rolling Stone*'s coverage and the significant, professional disagreements among the pages of the *Journal of Gay and Lesbian
Psychotherapy* are not, in themselves, the most alarming issues. Instead,
this responsibility might more productively take the form of waiting or,
as Derrida might put it, of letting be. This does not have to be an idle
waiting; in the meantime, we might work toward promoting more
savvy forms of "discourse literacy" for gay men and those who care

about them. Such literacy might begin with revitalizing the distinction between barebacking and bug chasing, not as different forms of perversion or separate diagnoses but as names we give ourselves in an attempt to comprehend behaviors and desires that, at the moment, exceed our powers of understanding and explanation.

NOTES

I would like to thank Evan Axelbank, Diane Cady, Camie Welch, Rose Ellen Lessy, and Fred Estabrook for their material and intellectual assistance with this essay.

1. See, for example, Brian K. Goodroad et al., "Bareback Sex and Gay Men: An HIV Prevention Failure," *Journal of the Association of Nurses in AIDS Care* 11, no. 6 (2000): 29–36.

2. Recent responses in the gay press to barebacking and bug chasing include Andrew Sullivan, "Sex- and Death-Crazed Gays Play Viral Russian Roulette!" Salon.com, January 24, 2003, http://www.salon.com/opinion/sullivan/2003/01/24/rolling/ (accessed April 4, 2004); and Eric Rofes, "Barebacking and the New AIDS Hysteria," *Seattle Stranger*, April 8, 1999, http://www.thestranger.com/1999-04-08/feature.html (accessed April 4, 2004).

3. Dan Savage, "Savage Love," *Seattle Stranger*, January 30, 2003, http://www.thestranger.com/2003-01-30/savage.html (accessed April 12, 2004); and Gregory A. Freeman, "In Search of Death," *Rolling Stone*, February 6, 2003, 44–8.

4. For an in-depth discussion of how cultural studies methodologies more generally, and Foucault's theories in particular, are applicable to the study of health, risk, and the health sciences, see John Tulloch and Deborah Lupton, *Television, AIDS, and Risk* (St Leonards, NSW, Australia: Allen and Unwin, 1997); and Lupton, *The Imperative of Health: Public Health and the Regulated Body* (Thousand Oaks, CA: Sage Publications, 1995). Lupton argues, for example, that "[j]ust as biomedical knowledges, discourses, and practices create their objects and fields of interest—disease, illnesses, patients, surgical techniques—the knowledges, discourses and practices of public health serve both to constitute and regulate such phenomena as 'normality,' 'risk,' and 'health'" (*Imperative*, 4).

5. Freeman, 44–8. Subsequent references are cited parenthetically in the text.

6. Several recent studies have attempted to catalog the reasons men engage in risky sex. See, for example, J. P. Cheuvront, "High-Risk Sexual Behavior in the Treatment of HIV-Negative Patients," *Journal of Gay and Lesbian Psychotherapy* 6, no. 37 (2002): 7–25 (subsequent references are cited parenthetically in the text); Mark Davis, "HIV Prevention Rationalities and Serostatus in the Risk Narratives of Gay Men," *Sexualities* 5, no. 3 (2002): 281–99; DeAnn K. Gauthier and Craig J. Forsyth, "Bareback Sex, Bug Chasers, and the Gift of Death," *Deviant Behavior: An Interdisciplinary Journal* 20, no. 1 (1999): 85–100; Goodroad et al.; Perry N. Halkitis and Jeffrey T. Parsons, "Intentional Unsafe Sex (Barebacking) among HIV-Positive Gay Men Who Seek Sexual Partners on the Internet," *AIDS Care* 15, no. 3 (2003): 367–78; Gordon Mansergh et al., "'Barebacking' in a Diverse Sample of Men Who Have Sex with Men," *AIDS* 16 (2002): 653–9; Troy Suarez and Jeffrey Miller, "Negotiating Risks in Context: A Perspective on Unprotected Anal Intercourse and Barebacking Among Men Who Have Sex with Men—Where Do We Go from Here?" *Archives of Sexual Behavior* 30, no. 3 (2001): 287–300; and Gust A. Yep et al., "The Case of 'Riding Bareback': Sexual Practices and the Paradoxes of Identity in the Era of AIDS," *Journal of Homosexuality* 42, no. 4 (2002): 1–14.

7. Harvey Fierstein, "The Culture of Disease," *New York Times*, July 31, 2003, A25; and Troy Suarez et al., "Selective Serotonin Reuptake Inhibitors as a Treatment for Sexual Compulsivity," in *Beyond Condoms: Alternative Approaches to HIV Prevention*, ed. Ann O'Leary (New York: Kluwer Academic/Plenum Publishers, 2002), 199–220.

8. Benoit Denizet-Lewis, "Double Lives on the Down Low," *New York Times Magazine*, August 3, 2003, 28.

9. Capitalizing the "O" in "Other" serves to emphasize another subject's separateness from one's own consciousness. Jacques Derrida and Emmanuel Levinas both write about the ethical and metaphysical problem and, indeed, the impossibility of ever fully recognizing the Other as fully separate. See Jacques Derrida, "Violence and Metaphysics: An Essay on the Thought of Emmanuel Levinas," in *Writing and Difference*, trans. Alan Bass (Chicago: University of Chicago Press, 1978), 79–153. Subsequent references are cited parenthetically in the text.

10. By way of explaining this rather perplexing claim, Derrida writes that "A Being without violence would be a Being which would occur outside the existent: nothing; nonhistory; nonoccurrence; nonphenomenality. A speech produced without the least violence would determine nothing, would say nothing, would offer nothing to the other; it would not be *history*, and it would *show* nothing . . ." (147, Derrida's italics).

11. Sullivan, "Sex- and Death-Crazed Gays."

12. "Discourse Analysis," in *The Bedford Glossary of Critical and Literary Terms*, ed. Ross Murfin and Supryia M. Ray, 2nd ed. (Boston: Bedford/St. Martin's, 2003), 114.

13. The blurring of barebacking into bug chasing might be read as a manifestation of so-called "sex panic" by some gay activists. Eric Rofes, in particular, has raised the question of whether or not gay men have become victims of a new sexual hysteria. See Eric Rofes, "Barebacking and the New AIDS Hysteria" and "The Emerging Sex Panic Targeting Gay Men" (lecture, National Gay and Lesbian Task Force Creating Change Conference, San Diego, CA, November 16, 1997), http://www.managingdesire.org/sexpanic/rofessexpanic.html (accessed April 12, 2004).

14. See Eric Vittinghoff et al., "Per-Contact Risk of Human Immunodeficiency Virus Transmission between Male Sexual Partners," *American Journal of Epidemiology* 150 (1999): 306–11. For other recent assessments of the risk of acquiring HIV associated with specific sexual activities, see Richard J. Wolitski and Bernard M. Branson, "'Gray Area Behaviors' and Partner Selection Strategies," in O'Leary, *Beyond Condoms : Alternative Approaches to HIV Prevention*, 173–98; Victor DeGruttola et al., "Infectiousness of HIV Between Male Homosexual Partners," *Journal of Clinical Epidemiology* 42, no. 9 (1989): 849–56; and John A. Jacquez et al., "Role of the Primary Infection in Epidemics of HIV Infection in Gay Cohorts," *Journal of Acquired Immune Deficiency Syndromes* 7, no. 11 (1994): 1169–84. While studies such as those cited here provide a quantitative baseline for understanding the overall infectivity of HIV in relation to specific sexual acts, recent studies have shown that other factors can increase a person's chance of both transmitting and becoming infected with HIV. Tears in mucous membranes are obvious sites for the transmission of HIV, and common sense suggests that internal tissues that form a barrier to infection can be disrupted by frequent intercourse. In addition, people with certain STDs are also at greater risk of infection. The work of M. C. Atkins et al. is particularly pertinent here: "Most HIV infections worldwide are acquired sexually, yet most coital episodes involving an infected partner do not result in acquisition of HIV. Acquisition of HIV must depend on both the volume of secretions transferred from the infected partner (donor) and the concentration of HIV present in the secretions. However, exposure alone to such a virus inoculum is clearly insufficient to ensure transmission. The coexistence of other sexually transmitted diseases in either the recipient or donor could potentially increase the risk of transmission by causing genital ulcers or by releasing inflammatory cytokines which increase HIV replication." See M. C. Atkins

et al., "Fluctuations of HIV Load in Semen of HIV Positive Patients with Newly Acquired Sexually Transmitted Diseases," *British Medical Journal* 313 (1996): 341–2. See also Timothy Schacker et al., "Frequent Recovery of HIV-1 from Genital Herpes Simplex Virus Lesions in HIV Infected Men," *JAMA* 280, no. 1 (1998): 61–6; Judith N. Wasserheit, "Epidemiological Synergy: Interrelationships between HIV Infection and Other Sexually Transmitted Diseases," *Sexually Transmitted Diseases* 19, no. 2 (1992): 61–77; and Myron S. Cohen, "Sexually Transmitted Diseases Enhance HIV Transmission: No Longer a Hypothesis," *Lancet* 351, no. 9119 (1998): 5–7.

15. Mark J. Blechner, "Intimacy, Pleasure, Risk, and Safety: Discussion of Cheuvront's 'High-Risk Sexual Behavior in the Treatment of HIV-Negative Patients,'" *Journal of Gay and Lesbian Psychotherapy* 6, no. 3 (2002): 27–33, 32. Subsequent references are cited parenthetically in the text.

16. Mansergh et al., 654.

17. While I cannot here fully elaborate on this formulation, there has been much work done in queer theory on what might be called the "politicization of the anus." See especially Leo Bersani, "Is the Rectum a Grave?" in *AIDS: Cultural Analysis/Cultural Activism*, ed. Douglas Crimp (Cambridge: MIT Press, 1988), 197–222; and Eve Kosofsky Sedgwick, "Is the Rectum Straight?: Identification and Identity in *The Wings of the Dove*," in *Tendencies* (Durham, NC: Duke University Press, 1993), 73–103. For a public-health perspective, see Gary Dowsett, "The Indeterminate Macro-Social: New Traps for Old Players in HIV/AIDS Social Research," *Culture, Health and Sexuality* 1, no. 1 (1999): 95–102, esp. 98.

18. Stephen Gendin, "They Shoot Barebackers, Don't They?" *POZ* 44 (1999): 48–51, 69; and Michael Scarce, "A Ride on the Wild Side," *POZ* 44 (1999): 52–5, 70–1. Subsequent references are cited parenthetically in the text.

19. Jack Felson, review of *They Shoot Horses, Don't They?* by Horace McCoy, amazon.com, June 10, 2002, http://www.amazon.com/exec/obidos/ASIN/185242401X/102-9048209-8486549 (accessed April 4, 2004).

20. Goodroad et al., 30.

21. Suarez and Miller, 289. See also, for other examples, Cheuvront, Davis, Gauthier and Forsyth, and Yep.

22. Steven Epstein, *Impure Science: AIDS, Activism, and the Politics of Knowledge* (Berkeley: University of California Press, 1996).

23. Gauthier and Forsyth, 96.

24. The claim was attributed to Dr. Bob Cabaj, director of Community Behavioral Health Services for San Francisco County, who denies having made it. See Seth Mnookin, "Is Rolling Stone's HIV Story Wildly Exaggerated?" *Newsweek* Web Exclusive, January 23, 2003, http://msnbc.msn.com/id/3668484 (accessed April 12, 2004); and Ellen Sorokin, "'Bug Chaser' AIDS Story Disputed," *Washington Times*, January, 24, 2003, http://www.washingtontimes.com (accessed April 12, 2004).

25. Louis P. Sheldon, "Bug Chasing and Barebacking: Homosexuals Go Looking for Death," Traditional Values Coalition Web site, January 28, 2003, http://traditionalvalues.org/modules.php?name=News&file=article&sid=717 (accessed April 5, 2004).

26. Sullivan writes all this in "Sex- and Death-Crazed Gays" while *also* describing the *Rolling Stone* article as "hysteria, wrapped in a homophobic and HIV-phobic wrapper."

27. Savage, "Savage Love."

28. The limitations of and backlash against early sex-safe messages have been widely discussed in public-health literature. Two particularly insightful studies of these failures are Walt Odets, *In the Shadow of the Epidemic: Being HIV-Negative in the Age of AIDS* (Durham, NC: Duke University Press, 1995); and Cindy Patton, *Fatal Advice: How Safe-Sex Education Went Wrong* (Durham, NC: Duke University Press, 1996).

29. For recent examples of work in this vein outside of the United States, see Davis and Dowsett.

30. O'Leary, *Beyond Condoms: Alternative Approaches to HIV Prevention*, xi.

31. Gauthier and Forsyth, 94.

32. For an overview of this process of medicalization, see Paula Bennett and Vernon A. Rosario II, eds., *Solitary Pleasures: The Historical, Literary, and Artistic Discourses of Autoeroticism* (New York: Routledge, 1995), 1–17.

33. Donna M. Orange, "High-Risk Behavior or High-Risk Systems? Discussion of Cheuvront's 'High-Risk Sexual Behavior in the Treatment of HIV-Negative Patients,'" *Journal of Gay and Lesbian Psychotherapy* 6, no. 3 (2002): 45–50. Subsequent references are cited parenthetically in the text.

34. Michael Scarce, "Bareback Sex: Implications for the Future of HIV Prevention," InSite Roundtable Discussion, University of California, San Francisco, May 1999. Transcript available online, http://hivinsite.ucsf.edu/InSite.jsp?doc=2098.418e (accessed April 5, 2004).

35. Rofes, "Barebacking and the New AIDS Hysteria."

36. Davis, 294.

37. Yep, 12.

38. Jacques Derrida, *The Gift of Death*, trans. David Wills (Chicago: University of Chicago Press, 1995), 25.

39. Marshall Forstein, "Commentary on Cheuvront's 'High-Risk Sexual Behavior in the Treatment of HIV-Negative Patients,'" *Journal of Gay and Lesbian Psychotherapy* 6, no. 3 (2002): 35–43, 36. Subsequent references are cited parenthetically in the text.

40. For more on the concept of performativity, see Judith Butler, *Gender Trouble: Feminism and the Subversion of Identity* (New York: Routledge, 1990); and Andrew Parker and Eve Kosofsky Sedgwick, *Performativity and Performance* (New York: Routledge, 1995), esp. 1–18.

41. Thus Steven F. Kruger, in his book *AIDS Narratives: Gender and Sexuality, Fiction and Science* (New York: Garland, 1996), sets out "to show the ways in which scientific discourses are in fact coopted for, implicated in, at the service of sexist, heterosexist, and racist representations" (4).

42. For an extended discussion of "exposure" as a critical imperative, see Eve Kosofsky Sedgwick, *Novel Gazing: Queer Readings in Fiction* (Durham, NC: Duke University Press, 1997).

"Without us all told": Paul Monette's Vigilant Witnessing to the AIDS Crisis

Lisa Diedrich

On October 22, 1986, Paul Monette's lover, Roger Horwitz, died of AIDS. "That is the only real date anymore," Monette writes, "casting its ice shadow over all the secular holidays lovers mark their calendars by."[1] In the year following Roger's death, Monette, himself HIV positive and up until then known (or not known as the case may be) as a writer of rather banal novels, earnest poetry, and film novelizations, would write two works, *Love Alone* and *Borrowed Time*, that bear both personal and public witness to the early days of the AIDS epidemic in the United States.[2] Before his own death of AIDS on February 10, 1995, Monette would write two autobiographical works, *Becoming a Man* (1992), which describes his torturous coming-out, and *Last Watch of the Night* (1994), a collection of "essays too personal and otherwise," that chronicle his continued witnessing to AIDS.[3] It is no small irony that AIDS both gave Monette his voice and mortally wounded him; his voice and his wound are inextricably bound to each other "as the condition of the possibility of telling" his story and the stories of others.[4]

The voice that emerges in Monette's writings on AIDS is an ethical voice; it is a voice of witness connected intimately to his experiences of loss, love, and mortality (his own and others). "I buy time with another story," Audre Lorde writes, but Monette understands that time cannot be bought but merely borrowed, implying a debt that casts its shadow on the future.[5] *Borrowed Time* opens with the jarring statement, "I don't know if I will live to finish this." Monette continues:

> Doubtless there's a streak of self-importance in such an assertion, but who's counting? Maybe it's just that I've watched too many sicken in a month and die by Christmas, so that a fatal sort of realism comforts me more than magic. All I know is this: The virus ticks in

me. And it doesn't care a whit about our categories—when is full-blown, what's AIDS-related, what is just sick and tired? No one has solved the puzzle of its timing. I take my drug from Tijuana twice a day. The very friends who tell me how vigorous I look, how well I seem, are the first to assure me of the imminent medical break-through. What they don't seem to understand is, I used up all my optimism keeping my friend alive. Now that he's gone, the cup of my own health is neither half full nor half empty. Just half. (1–2)

Monette did live to finish the book, but is there something more, beyond the book, that he senses he will not live to finish, that cannot be finished in language, that cannot be fully told? When he writes that, "the cup of my own health is neither half full nor half empty. Just half," Monette attempts to explain his predicament. The "just half," in Monette's formulation, resists any easy interpretation which would reduce this to a story of hope ("half full") or a story of hopelessness ("half empty"). Monette's work is about the absolute necessity of telling of death (the death of Roger in the past, the death of Paul himself in the future, and the epidemic of deaths from AIDS in the past, present, and future) as well as the impossibility of comprehending the meaning of death. In order to show the magnitude of both a single death and countless deaths, Monette returns again and again to personal and political scenes of loss, but also, importantly, to personal and political scenes of love. He explores different genres—memoir, poetry, essay, and fable—in order to find a suitable form.[6] What he discovers in this exploration of form, and the reader discovers in reading his work, however, is that there is no form particularly suited to what he urgently needs to say. Rather, his work achieves its emotional poignancy through the conflict between the urgency of Monette's witnessing and the inadequacy of the literary form to convey his message.

In the influential early collection of AIDS criticism, *Writing AIDS*, several authors read Monette's work as exemplary of particular forms of AIDS writing. John M. Clum calls Monette the "paradigmatic writer in this new barren land of displacement, pain, and loss" and "the bard of AIDS."[7] In his comparison between two modes of AIDS writing, which he calls immersive and counterimmersive, Joseph Cady reads Monette as a classic example of the immersive mode. According to Cady, immersive writing attempts to confront the denial surrounding AIDS by thrusting the reader "into a direct imaginative confrontation with the special horrors of AIDS."[8] Counterimmersive writing, on the other hand, portrays AIDS tangentially. Cady favors the immersive form because he fears that counterimmersive writing "runs the risk of ultimately collaborating with the larger cultural denial of the disease."[9] Finally, Timothy F. Murphy's essay, "Testimony," provides an important discussion of AIDS writers, including Monette, who write about the epidemic in the testimonial form. Murphy defines testimony as "witness in front of an indifferent world about the worth and merit of persons. And thus one writes, for the world unconvinced, that someone was here and that, death notwithstanding, a presence remains."[10]

My essay seeks to build on the AIDS criticism of Murphy and others by reading Monette in relation to theories of witnessing that have developed roughly concurrently with the AIDS crisis. While I am aware that there is a large body of literary critical work on writings about AIDS in general and Monette's work in particular, my approach diverges somewhat from a conventional literary critical reading of Monette's work toward a more phenomenological examination of its philosophical grounding. As with most of my work on the literature of AIDS, I seek not only to read such literature through contemporary theories of subjectivity and the body but also to read those theories through the event and experience of AIDS as described in literature. Thus I will read Monette's work along with and through the work of the contemporary feminist philosopher Kelly Oliver. All of Oliver's work asks questions about the relationship between subjectivity and ethics and, in doing so, engages with a wide range of nineteenth- and twentieth- century continental philosophers, including Friedrich Nietzsche, Jacques Derrida, Jacques Lacan, Luce Irigaray, and Julia Kristeva.

In her most recent work, *Witnessing: Beyond Recognition*, Oliver articulates a theory of witnessing that draws on and extends recent philosophical work on recognition as the basis for subjectivity, as well as psychoanalytic-influenced trauma theory, especially as articulated by literary theorist Shoshana Felman and psychoanalyst Dori Laub in their influential book *Testimony: Crisis of Witnessing in Literature, Psychoanalysis, and History* and historian Dominick LaCapra in *Representing the Holocaust: History, Theory, Trauma*.[11] Trauma theorists like Felman, Laub, LaCapra, Cathy Caruth, Lawrence Langer, and Maurice Blanchot have attempted to understand the relationship between trauma and experience and the ways that certain traumatic experiences are given voice in written and oral testimony.[12] Much of this theory has emerged out of an analysis of experiences of extreme violence, such as occurred during the Holocaust and other wartime events, but less has been written about illness as a traumatic event that, like violence, may be both necessary and difficult to witness. In her edited collection, *Trauma:*

Explorations in Memory, Caruth includes an interview with AIDS activists and cultural critics Gregg Bordowitz, Douglas Crimp, and Laura Pinsky, in which she asks them to discuss the ways in which the AIDS crisis can be viewed as trauma, which she defines as "a memory that one cannot integrate into one's own experience, and as a catastrophic knowledge that one cannot communicate to others."[13] In this paper, I want to pose a question similar to Caruth's and explore the answer through Monette's writings on AIDS and Oliver's theory of witnessing. How does Monette's work—in both its content and its multiple forms—demonstrate what Oliver, in *Witnessing: Beyond Recognition,* calls the "paradox of the eyewitness," which, as she describes it, is the "paradox between the necessity and impossibility of testimony"?[14]

In *Witnessing,* Oliver notes that the word "witnessing" has a double meaning: it means both "*eyewitness* testimony based on first-hand knowledge . . . and *bearing witness* [to others] to something beyond recognition that can't be seen" (16, Oliver's italics). The practice of witnessing, then, requires that we cultivate our "response-ability," in Oliver's terminology, to those things that we both see and do not see, hear and do not hear, and know and do not know. For Oliver, "[t]o serve subjectivity, and therefore humanity, we must be vigilant in our attempts to continually open and reopen the possibility of response" (19). This openness to the possibility of response is a means by which we might, as Monette attempts to do, tell both personal and political stories of loss and love that surround the experience of AIDS. In her philosophical investigations into the practices of witnessing, Oliver is concerned with the possibilities engendered in "working-through the trauma of oppression necessary to personal and political transformation" (85).

How does one become a responsible witness in Oliver's terms, and what kinds of personal and political transformations are enacted by this sort of witnessing? We, the readers of Monette's work, are also implicated in this process of witnessing; we too must cultivate our response-ability through our reading (at the very least) to those whom our society, in the age of AIDS, has made "other." Where AIDS is concerned, bodies have been devalued and "abjected" (reduced to vectors of disease and dehumanized) not just because of the way in which they are perceived as particular sexual bodies but also because of the way in which they are perceived as particular racial and national bodies. In his work, however, Monette is primarily concerned with the abjection of the gay body and love and/or sexuality between men. Therefore this will be the focus of my paper.[15] The paper is organized around three key terms in Oliver's work—history, vigilance, and working-through—and delineates her use of these terms and their place within an ethics and aesthetics of witnessing as performed in Monette's work on AIDS.

History

Drawing, in *Witnessing*, on the psychoanalytic work of Felman and Laub on Holocaust testimony, Oliver is concerned less with the historical accuracy of testimony than with the possibility that the "performance of testimony says more than the witness knows" (86). Such is the case in Monette's testimonies to the AIDS crisis; his AIDS writing not only entails what he knows about this illness and the process of learning about it and the death it brings, but it also reveals everything that he does not know, cannot know, and even refuses to know. Monette's work performs what Laub describes as the "*discovery* of knowledge—its evolution, and its very *happening*."[16] His opening sentence in *Borrowed Time*—"I don't know if I will live to finish this"—is only the beginning of a chronicle of knowing and not knowing, of certainty and uncertainty, of recognition and lack of recognition. The crisis of AIDS is, in other words, an epistemological crisis as well as an ontological crisis. Monette's writing is an attempt to describe the impossible position of having both too little knowledge (to prevent or treat this disease) and too much knowledge (of the fact of death: Roger's, his own, and, in the beginning at least, seemingly everyone who is infected).

One reason, perhaps, that Monette does not know if he will live to "finish this" is that he does not even know where to begin. Although he knows that, at the time of his writing *Borrowed Time*, it is the "seventh year of the calamity," he does not know when and where it all began (2). The opening chapter of this text attempts—and fails—to pinpoint when he, and everyone else in the gay community in Los Angeles, began to know something. There are signs: a note in his diary in December 1981 about "ambiguous reports of a 'gay cancer,'" but, Monette admits, at that time, "I know I didn't have the slightest picture of the thing" (3). What is this thing that is imperceptible (and, for us, unreadable), even from a position seven years into it? How can we begin to look at this thing, begin to see it, begin to read it, begin to know it? As Oliver notes in *Witnessing*, with regard to victims of oppression in general, but which might be applied to the experience of people with AIDS in particular, what one must seek is not merely "visibility and recognition"; one must also "witness to horrors beyond recognition" (8). What would a history of this witnessing look, sound, and feel like? In his writing, Monette attempts to give this history, which is a history of the practices of witnessing as much as a history of AIDS among gay men in the United States.

The difficulty for Monette, of course, is that he is *in it*: in the thing, the calamity, not outside of it, or past it. Oliver asserts, again in *Witnessing*, that "it is impossible to testify from inside" a traumatic event, because the trauma possesses us so entirely that there is no outside of the event to which we might relate our experience. And yet, Oliver continues, "in order to reestablish subjectivity and in order to demand justice, it is necessary to bear witness to the inarticulate experience of the inside" (90). Bearing witness to the inarticulate experience of the inside of AIDS is Monette's task, and it is an infinite task. His work attempts to give form to this inside that lacks parameters either in time or space.[17] Monette writes in *Borrowed Time* that when he first read reports of a "gay cancer" in 1981, he thought at the time, "How is this not me?" (3) This is a strange question; it is, in fact, grammatically strange, but more importantly it reveals *a grammar of estrangement*. That is, it reveals a knowledge of the self that is founded upon a failure of knowledge of the self. "How is this not me?" is a question, moreover, that structures all of Monette's writings on AIDS and, I contend, most narratives that attempt to describe the experience of illness or trauma from the inside. It is also a question that does not close off but, rather, opens up the possibility of response. And it is a question that not only reveals how one experiences AIDS in particular or illness in general but also suggests a theory of subjectivity that resonates with Oliver's.

Other theories of subjectivity place the annihilation of difference at their center, and they understand identity as a fixed and stable category of being. Oliver, however, in her book *Family Values: Subjects between Nature and Culture*, maintains that differences—how is this not me?—are what motivate a person to "try to move out of myself towards you in order to commune with that which ultimately I can never know."[18] She continues: "[I]t is through our relationship and our *differences* that I can begin to see something of myself. . . . We experience our lives as flux and flow, full of surprises even to ourselves."[19] Monette's question is significant simply because it is a question. When he asks, "How is this not me?" he reveals the possibility of surprise in his attempts to answer that question. If this is not me, then who is it, or what is it, and who am I? In the moment of estrangement

Monette is unable to separate himself from the "not me," and his question opens up the possibility of encountering the "not me" in others as well as himself. Moreover, the movement "out of myself towards you in order to commune with that which ultimately I can never know" not only occurs across the spaces between bodies and between body and world but also across time. Our experiences of ourselves are not contained or containable because, simply put, we experience them in time, and our knowledge of those experiences is always subject to time. We can begin to make this movement outside of ourselves toward difference when we acknowledge the possibility that *in time the not me might become me*, or, more simply, *in time the not me is me, is who I am*. Such a movement outside of oneself toward the other or the not me requires what Oliver calls vigilance, the next of my key terms from her work.

Vigilance

In a reading of Freud's *Beyond the Pleasure Principle*, Cathy Caruth notes that "[w]hat Freud encounters in the traumatic neurosis is not the reaction to any horrible event but, rather, the peculiar and perplexing experience of survival."[20] According to Caruth's reading of Freud, trauma is not simply the experience of a traumatic event itself, but the survival of that event; that is, trauma is not only a "crisis of death" but also a "crisis of life."[21] Survival is imbued with anguish not only because of one's traumatic encounter with death but because one's own survival "is inseparably identified with victims who did not survive."[22] In his writing, Monette demonstrates this peculiar and perplexing experience of survival in his vigilant witnessing to all those who did not survive. For Monette, the victims of AIDS in the early years of the epidemic include not only lovers and friends but also countless others he will never know and whose voices—unlike his own—are now lost to us. Monette's own survival (for a time) makes him feel responsible for those countless lost voices, and his writing attempts to enact this response-ability, at the same time showing the immense difficulty of such response-ability.

In *Borrowed Time*, we learn that Monette misses Roger's actual death; he is sleeping "curled up in Roger's bed" when the call comes from UCLA Medical Center. For Monette, sleeping does not avoid the fact of Roger's death so much as avoid the fact of his own survival: "waking," Monette writes, "teaches you pain" (342). *Borrowed Time* ends with Monette "[p]utting off as long as I could the desolate waking to

life alone—this calamity that is all mine, that will not end till I do"
(342). In the poem "Dreaming of You" from *Love Alone* Monette
elaborates further on the ways in which he attempts to hold at bay the
nightmare of waking to his own survival, for in sleep and dreams
Roger returns to him:

> give me night
> give me more of it I wish to be an expert
> on darkness and all it conjures wish to sleep-
> walk with you no matter how queer a scene
> the crooked synapses of my brain cast us in
> a dream is never the one line long enough
> what's even worse we can't go walking after
> to watch from the canyon rim while the west
> burns midnight they are brief they are shadows
> they evaporate I wake I forget them
> but if they're all I have then let them come
> cascading. . . .
>
> (57, lines 44 55)

Sleep and dreams for Monette do not, however, "come cascading." In
fact, in the essay "Sleeping Under a Tree" from *Last Watch of the Night*,
we learn that Monette suffers from acute insomnia, a condition which
he presciently (or so it would seem) develops the night before Roger's
diagnosis. Monette's insomnia, in its timing and manifestation, exemplifies what Oliver, following Emmanuel Levinas, defines as vigilance. As
with the term "witnessing," Oliver, in *Witnessing*, notes two "radically
different" meanings for vigilance: "both observing or keeping watch
and responding to something beyond your own control" (134).

This double meaning of vigilance, as with the double meaning of
witnessing, relies on an understanding of the Levinasian concepts of
"beyond intentionality" and "wakefulness." On the one hand, the
alertness and watchfulness of vigilance is "something that one intends
to do," and on the other hand, it is "beyond intentionality," in Levinas's
terms, and "appears as a response to something or someone beyond
one's self," Oliver writes in *Witnessing* (134). In Monette's case, while
Roger is alive, his wakefulness has a purpose: he watches over Roger's
much-needed slumber, preparing dosages at intervals throughout the
night and feeding them to Roger "without really waking him up."[23] In

the week of his death, Roger tells his doctor, "'I'm sleeping for everyone now.'" The doctor understands his remark as a sign of "serious brain involvement," but Monette writes in *Last Watch* that he thinks the remark is "piercingly wise and tender," and believes that Roger is "sleeping *le sommeil du juste*—the sleep of the just—for all the rest of us, pursued day and night by our compromises with nightmares" (252, Monette's italics). After Roger's death, Monette understands his role as the obverse of Roger's sleep for the just: "*I'm having insomnia for everyone now*" (252, Monette's italics). Monette's nocturnal vigils, to use Oliver's terms from *Witnessing*, are "not the vigilance of a self-possessed watchfulness but the vigilance of a self opened onto otherness itself" (134). Monette's "self opened onto otherness itself" is the price he must pay for his own survival; it is, as he describes it, an exile into a "parallel universe, lunar and featureless" where all he desires is sleep.[24] But sleep, like death, is the very thing that eludes him.

The call around 6 AM that awakens Monette after Roger's death is repeated again four years later when another call comes, this time just after 4 AM, to say that Stephen, Monette's second lover to die of AIDS, is gone as well. "I think I've never stopped hearing that twice-tolled ring in the night," Monette admits in the essay "Sleeping Under a Tree, from *Last Watch*." He describes waking almost every night around 4 AM (having drifted off only an hour or so before) "in a panic, still waiting for that call. Sometimes the ghost of an echo, as if I've already missed it" (244). The call announces death, but he always misses it, hearing only "the ghost of an echo," which announces not death, but survival, and what Oliver, in *Witnessing*, describes as the "demands of otherness" (134). The vision of hope that sustains Monette and keeps him awake and writing until his own death comes in a dream he has while napping with Roger at the mouth of a secluded cave in Hawaii. In "Sleeping Under a Tree," Monette dreams of Kollau the Leper, who led a resistance movement against the American troops that sought to transport a group of lepers to a colony at Molokai. The American gunboats were unable to break the lepers' resistance, and eventually the lepers were allowed to stay put and create, what Monette calls, an "outpost of Eden and a tribe at peace" (260). The "memory of the dream encounter" becomes a touchstone for Monette, and he understands his vigilance, his determination to keep watch physically through his insomnia and figuratively in his writing, as the means by which he might create another outpost of Eden and bring peace to another tribe of others (261). Monette is the night watchman of his tribe of people with AIDS, and, as he tells his readers in "Sleeping Under a Tree," he will sleep only when he is dead.

Monette reveals over and over that the trauma of Roger's death is also the trauma of his own awakening to survival and the ethical imperative that is inherent to that traumatic awakening. In the poem "Readiness," which appears in *Love Alone*, Monette considers suicide—"a cocked .32 will do in a pinch"—but admits, "I'm not half ready to leave us here / without us all told" (14, lines 61, 63–4). The odd locution of this sentence points again to a death that is always missed, yet still somehow must be recorded. The sentence also points to suicide as a sure means to avoid the response-ability of witnessing and the demands of otherness. In *Facing It*, Ross Chambers presents AIDS writing as an alternative—and the more difficult alternative, he believes—to suicide, which he describes as an "easier, and so tempting but ultimately unacceptable solution."[25] One must face death first as the appealing possibility of suicide, according to Chambers, before one can face death again "in the form of living with, and dying, of AIDS."[26]

In the poem "The Very Same" from his collection of poetry, *Love Alone*, Monette describes a moment just before Roger's death in which Roger, mostly blind, "sees" Monette come into his hospital room and says, *"But we're the same person / when did that happen"* (20, lines 33–4, Monette's italics). Roger's blindness is a form of seeing that entails more than vision. By "seeing" Paul as the same person as himself when he is blind and dying, Roger calls into question Monette's subjectivity. In doing so, he forces Monette to see himself from the vantage point of the other, expose himself to the other, and render account. "I had a self myself / once but he died," Monette declares in the poem "Manifesto," and while it may be that that self died along with Roger, it may also be that that self died in Roger's blind vision of sameness that, paradoxically, requires Monette to remain open to the demands of otherness (41, lines 69–70). This doubling—this death in life—that makes demands on Monette is apparent as well in the poem "Half Life," in which Monette grieves:

I get up and half of me doesn't
work I drag me like a broken wing my good
eye sees flesh and green the dead eye an X-
ray gaping at skeletons. . . .

                                                            (16, lines 10-13)

Monette sees through both eyes—good and dead—and his writing in "Half Life" presents both visions—flesh and green and skeletons. When Monette is told after Roger's death that it is *"time to turn / the page,"* to move past Roger's death, he retorts: "BUT THIS *IS* MY PAGE IT

CANNOT BE TURNED" (20, lines 3–4, 9, Monette's italics). Monette's work can be distilled into a single page that cannot be turned and must be filled with Roger and Paul's "growing interchangeability," until they are both all told (21, line 40).

Monette's survival gives him an ethical responsibility to bear witness not only to Roger's death and his own but also to the death of a generation as well. He admits in *Borrowed Time*, "I can't think of almost any moment of October [the month of Roger's death] without feeling helpless, like flinching in the glare of the final air burst. But how was I to know? Then I knew nothing about death, and now I know everything short of my own" (323). This knowledge is, paradoxically, both the impetus for and the impossibility of witnessing. Monette attempts, in *Borrowed Time*, to explain the paradox:

> It's like I died, and I didn't die. We are here, and we love each other, and now I have to find some work. Sentence by sentence, nothing by nothing, even if I can't sing. Then hum a few bars at least. Whistle a bit in the dark. We cannot all go down to defeat and darkness, we have to say we have been here. (129)

"Sentence by sentence, nothing by nothing . . . we have to say we have been here." Both the sentences and the nothing are part of the knowledge and must also be part of the vigilant witnessing. Monette must find work that testifies to those who have been here and are now gone and that testifies to love that is not perceived as such by the larger society. By humming a few bars and whistling in the darkness to say, "We have been here and we have loved each other," Monette counters what Oliver calls in *Between the Psyche and the Social: Psychoanalytic Social Theory* the "double alienation" of oppression, which "results not just from finding yourself in a world of ready-made meanings [which Oliver calls existential alienation] but from finding yourself there as one who has been denied the possibility of meaning making or making meaning your own without at the same time denying your own subjectivity."[27]

But when we say we have been *here* and that we have loved each other, Monette despairs, will anyone *hear* and understand? Will there be future witnessing? The challenge for Monette as well as for us—as readers and as witnesses—is not only to tell but to listen; that is, to grasp what Oliver terms in *Witnessing* as "the unseen in vision and the unspoken in speech" (2). What is demanded of the readers of AIDS narratives, then, is a "new kind of listening, the witnessing, precisely, *of impossibility*."[28]

Working-through

What this new kind of listening might be, as embodied by Monette and as practiced in his writing, is theorized by Oliver in her delineation of—or perhaps, more appropriately, her working-through of—Freud's concept of working-through. In the poem "Three Rings" from *Love Alone* and again in *Borrowed Time* and yet again in the essay "3275" from *Last Watch of the Night*, Monette returns to two scenes. His generic searches are attempts to make language and meaning say what he needs to say, despite, or indeed because of, the double alienation that attaches to the experience of AIDS. What these scenes, and Monette's attempts to represent them, show is working-through as an ethical theory and practice. In *Witnessing* Oliver writes, "'Working-through' is a profoundly ethical operation insofar as it forces us not only to acknowledge our relations and obligations to others—that is, the ethical foundations of subjectivity—but also thereby to transform those relations into more ethical relations through which we love or at least respect others rather than subordinate or kill them" (68–9). Working-through, for Monette, will require that he bear witness—that he "love or at least respect others"—not just in and through language but also in and through his body, an experience which he then must attempt to render into language.

Monette describes such a process when he visits Roger's grave ten weeks after his death. "3275" is the number of Roger's grave, and it is also, as we realize at the end of the essay entitled "3275," the number of Monette's grave as well. Both Roger Horwitz and Paul Monette, then, are inscribed not only in Monette's writing but also in the inscriptions marking their grave. In "3275" and in the poem "Three Rings," Monette tells of a visit to Roger's grave in which he buries in the grass a Zuni ring he has bought for Roger on a trip to New Mexico. After Monette buries the ring, he begins to moan, ventriloquizing Roger's own moaning in the hospital ten weeks before:

suddenly I'm moaning out loud
this very specific moan the echo of you
when I walked in the last day a horn sound
that knifes me still . . .

(31, lines 87–90)

. . . .
the moaning wouldn't go away so the day of
the rings I mimicked you ventriloquizing

your last sound desolate as a sea-bell
trying to figure what the hurt was where
had we disappeared to then I froze mid-moan
saw it all in a blaze YOU WERE CALLING ME.

(32, lines 103–8)

And from "3275":

Now ten weeks later, a stillborn year before me, I finally understand that the bleating sound on that last day was Roger calling my name. Through the pounding in his head, the blindness and the paralysis, all his bodily functions out of control, he had somehow heard me come in. Had waited. And once I understood that, I went mad. My moaning rose to a siren pitch, and I clawed at the grass that covered him. Possessed with a fury to dig the six feet down and tear open the lid and clasp him to me, whatever was left. I don't even know what stopped me—exhaustion, I guess, the utter meaninglessness of anything anymore. (102)

I have quoted at length from these passages in order to give the reader a sense of the repetition of the scene both in Monette's life and in his writing. By mimicking Roger's moan, he embodies that moan; in his performance of the moan, it possesses him. He hears it not only with his ears and his brain, but with the tissues of his body; he becomes, in the words of Lawrence Langer, an "active hearer."[29]

His understanding is delayed, but even as he records the moment again and again in his work, he does not—cannot—record the process of that understanding in words. The moan is in excess of what can be understood in language, but at the same time it must be brought to language in order that it may be heard:

I didn't know Death
had reached your lips muscles gone words dispersed
still you moaned my name so ancient wild and
lonely it took ten weeks to reach me now
I hear each melancholy wail a roar like
fallen lions holding on by your fingertips
till I arrived for how many drowning hours
to say *Goodbye I love you* all in my name.[30]

(32, lines 109–16, Monette's italics)

The moan is something greater than speech; it is the demand of otherness made across time and space. It becomes Monette's weather and compass, giving his work both its essence and its direction. Furthermore, it is his name. The moan becomes Monette, and he it, and in this way it leaps across bodies and time. In the scene Monette describes, emotions and affects migrate or radiate between human beings, not just through space but through time, from Roger to Paul and beyond Paul to his readers. At the grave, Monette's moaning and digging are an attempt to get closer to Roger's death but also to experience his (Monette's) own dying, his own burial, his own moment—an interminable moment, a moment outside of time—beyond the limit of language and knowledge.

In the working-through of this scene and in various forms of writing, Monette reveals that, still, this moment is beyond the recognition that the "hearing" of his name implies. To say that he finally and fully understands Roger's moan—that, in the grave scene, he grasps it—feels like consolation for a moment that seems to resist just such consolation. Monette needs to represent Roger's moan in order to recuperate something he has missed and will always miss. He projects onto Roger's moan his own needs, but he also shows in that moment that he is saying more than he knows, doing more than he intended. Roger's death is a death that only Roger can experience. Monette is always going to be too late; he will always miss the call of otherness. He could not be a part of Roger's death because death is about both the absolute aloneness of the person who dies and the absolute aloneness of the person who survives. There is, therefore, in this moment of the moan a need that is never met. The performance of the moan, in other words, says more than Monette's recognition of his name implies. Monette's interpretation of Roger's moan as his name is a need to contain the force of that which is beyond language.

By making such an assertion, I do not mean to imply that Monette is somehow wrong or mistaken in hearing his name in the moan. What I do want to suggest, however, is that in the witnessing of something beyond recognition, Monette transmits not only the fact of the moan in narrative and the translation of the moan into his name but also the affective force of the moan as well. We, the readers, must attempt to hear both the address and the affective force of the address; for through our response-ability to both the address and the affective force of the address, we keep open the possibility of future witnessing. And keeping open the possibility of future witnessing is, finally, about love, another key term in Oliver's work that is a crucial aspect of a theory—and a practice—of subjectivity beyond recognition. In *Witnessing* Oliver writes, "To love is to bear witness to the process of witnessing that gives us the power to be, together. And being together is the chaotic adventure of subjectivity" (224). Monette's testimony to the experience of AIDS reveals this chaotic adventure of subjectivity in his performance of being together—with Roger, with countless others who have lived with and died of AIDS, and with his readers (even beyond Monette's own death of AIDS)—across space and time.

NOTES

1. Paul Monette, *Borrowed Time: An AIDS Memoir* (New York: Harcourt Brace and Company, 1988), 2. Subsequent references are cited parenthetically in the text.

2. Paul Monette, *Love Alone: Eighteen Elegies for Rog* (New York: St. Martin's Press, 1988). Subsequent references to Monette's poetry refer to this collection, with page and line numbers cited parenthetically in the text.

3. Paul Monette, *Becoming a Man: Half a Life Story* (New York: Harcourt Brace Jovanovich, 1992); and *Last Watch of the Night: Essays Too Personal and Otherwise* (New York: Harcourt Brace and Company, 1994).

4. Carol Jacobs, *Telling Time: Lévi-Strauss, Ford, Lessing, Benjamin, de Man, Wordsworth, Rilke* (Baltimore: Johns Hopkins University Press, 1993), 3.

5. Audre Lorde, "There Are No Honest Poems about Dead Women," *The Collected Poems of Audre Lorde* (New York: W. W. Norton, 1997), 409, line 15.

6. Monette works with fable in the posthumously published *Sanctuary: A Tale of Life in the Woods* (New York: Scribner, 1997).

7. John M. Clum, "'And Once I Had It All': AIDS Narratives and Memories of an American Dream," in *Writing AIDS: Gay Literature, Language, and Analysis*, ed. Timothy F. Murphy and Suzanne Poirier, 200–24 (New York: Columbia University Press, 1993), 209 and 210.

8. Joseph Cady, "Immersive and Counterimmersive Writing about AIDS: The Achievement of Paul Monette's *Love Alone*," in Murphy and Poirier, *Writing AIDS: Gay Literature, Language, and Analysis*, 244–64, 244.

9. Ibid., 261.

10. Timothy F. Murphy, "Testimony," in Murphy and Poirier, *Writing AIDS: Gay Literature, Language, and Analysis*, 306–20, 317.

11. Shoshana Felman and Dori Laub, *Testimony: Crises of Witnessing in Literature, Psychoanalysis, and History* (New York: Routledge, 1992); and Dominick LaCapra, *Representing the Holocaust: History, Theory, Trauma* (Ithaca, NY: Cornell University Press, 1994).

12. Cathy Caruth, *Unclaimed Experience: Trauma, Narrative, and History* (Baltimore: Johns Hopkins University Press, 1996); Caruth, ed., *Trauma: Explorations in Memory* (Baltimore: Johns Hopkins University Press, 1995); and Maurice Blanchot, *The Writing of the Disaster*, trans. Ann Smock (Lincoln: University of Nebraska Press, 1995).

13. Cathy Caruth and Thomas Keenan, "'The AIDS Crisis Is Not Over': A Conversation with Gregg Bordowitz, Douglas Crimp, and Laura Pinsky," in Caruth, *Trauma*, 256–71, 256.

14. Kelly Oliver, *Witnessing: Beyond Recognition* (Minneapolis: University of Minnesota Press, 2001), 86. Subsequent references are cited parenthetically in the text.

15. For a discussion of Monette's *Becoming a Man*, along with Audre Lorde's *The Cancer Journals*, in relation to abjection, as theorized by Judith Butler and Julia Kristeva, see Allison Kimmich, "Writing the Body: From Abject to Subject," *A/B: Auto/Biography* 13, no. 2 (1998): 223–4.

16. Felman and Laub, 62 (Felman and Laub's italics).

17. Joseph Cady notes that in his collection of poems, *Love Alone*, "Monette matches his harrowing content with a harrowing style by upsetting every conventional expectation of order an audience might bring to the text" (249). In the poem "Three Rings," Monette captures an image of trauma: "why the world though stopped like a car wreck keeps doubling back" (*Love Alone*, 33). Cady understands that "Monette incarnates this total 'wrecking' of his world in a thoroughly 'wrecked' form, designed to subject his readers to an immersive 'wrecking' in turn" (250).

18. Kelly Oliver, *Family Values: Subjects between Nature and Culture* (New York: Routledge, 1997), 96.

19. Ibid., 96–7 (my italics).

20. Caruth, *Unclaimed Experience*, 60.

21. Ibid., 7.

22. Lawrence L. Langer, *Holocaust Testimonies: The Ruins of Memory* (New Haven: Yale University Press, 1991), 75.

23. Monette, *Last Watch*, 243. Subsequent references are cited parenthetically in the text.

24. The trope of exile into a parallel universe recurs in Monette's work. In an attempt to describe this sense of "radical separateness" and liminality that the experience of AIDS affords, Monette, throughout *Borrowed Time*, characterizes the experience of having AIDS as an exile "on the moon." For a discussion of the trope of exile, see Anne Hunsaker Hawkins, *Reconstructing Illness: Studies in Pathography* (West Lafayette, IN: Purdue University Press, 1993), 81.

25. Ross Chambers, *Facing It: AIDS Diaries and the Death of the Author* (Ann Arbor: University of Michigan Press, 1998), 24.

26. Ibid.

27. Kelly Oliver, "Psychic Space and Social Melancholy" in *Between the Psyche and the Social: Psychoanalytic Social Theory*, ed. Kelly Oliver and Steve Edwin, 49–65 (Lanham, MD: Rowman and Littlefield, 2002), 56.

28. Caruth, *Trauma*, 10 (Caruth's italics).

29. Langer, 21.

30. In *The Writing of the Disaster*, Maurice Blanchot writes that "the cry tends to exceed all language, even if it lends itself to recuperation as language effect. It is both sudden and patient; it has the suddenness of the interminable torment which is always over already. The patience of the cry: it does not simply come to a halt, reduced to nonsense, yet it does remain outside of sense—a meaning infinitely suspended, decried, decipherable-indecipherable" (51).

Response to Section II:
Dis-sexuality
Sexuality and Dis-Sexuality in the International Regime of Human Rights

Sidonie Smith

I come to the three essays in this section on Sexuality/Dis-Sexuality with my own particular question: How does sexuality and dis-sexuality play in the contemporary regime of human rights with regard to the identities and differences that regime sets in motion? Having just coauthored (with Kay Schaffer) a book on human rights and narrated lives, I am particularly interested in examining the issues that arise when we situate cultural projects within a human-rights framework and within the intersections of rights politics and narrative practices. The following comments do not so much attempt to engage the arguments of these essays as to raise questions about our understanding of the meanings assigned to sexuality and dis-sexuality at this historical conjuncture.

Sue Sun Yom takes us back to the late 1960s for an examination of the politics of representation in the Vietnam War-era sex-education film *Where the Girls Are—VD in Southeast Asia*. Yom teases out the gendered logics of representation in the management of venereal disease: the threatening and exotic prostitutes of Vietnam, the innocent and faithful young woman left behind in the American home, and the gullible serviceman caught between the snares of excessive sexual excitement and his military duties. *Girls* exposes how sexual predation became another battleground in America's engagement with the constantly shifting grounds of a guerilla war. (It is tempting to interpret *Girls* as an explanatory exposé of the increasing impossibility of prosecuting a successful war in Southeast Asia.) Even in his search for rest and relaxation, the American soldier confronted an "enemy" out to confuse and contaminate him. In the logic of the film, and the logic of a military regime concerned with maximizing the readiness and fighting efficiency of its troops, the sexualized military body is paradoxically fit and unfit, dominant and yet victimized by a maelstrom of desire. Paradoxically, then, in this zone of "hetero-national masculinity," the film must position the United States soldier as "weak" before the onslaught of the inscrutable, wily, and feminine "other," in relation to whom he becomes a "victim."[1]

Yom suggests that the production of Girls marks a transition to a stance of "cautious engagement" with the economic realities of the militarized sex industry, but that it also projects the enemy's women as objects of contemptuous appropriation and the sex-entertainment industry as a naturalized business of war. And what of the young women enlisted by the early venture capitalists of the Southeast Asian sex trade? The "girls" in Girls do not speak, cannot speak. The Vietnamese women in the sex trade of the 1960s were unable to tell their stories (though a romanticized story would be told about them a decade later when Miss Saigon hit the stage with its droning helicopter and Madame Butterfly tropes). At that point, there was no discourse in the United States or elsewhere through which to understand the profiteering on the sex trade and sex tourism in Southeast Asia as state-sanctioned, organized exploitation of and violence against women, especially impoverished women. Some thirty-five years later, one wonders about the stories that haunt the film's narrative, stories which depict the unspoken cultural subordination of women and their bodies within Vietnamese society and within the zone of United States imperialism and war making.

Twenty-five years after Girls was shot, a pre–Vietnam War generation of women with experience in organized prostitution around military bases began to speak out publicly about their horrifying pasts. They too were enlisted in the sex trade attached to wartime; they too were enlisted in the project of keeping military men fit for battle. They also come from Southeast Asia and jugun ianfu (military comfort women) is the euphemistic term used to refer to them. When the spread of venereal disease threatened the preparedness of the Japanese Imperial Army during the Pacific War, the military hired sex brokers to recruit native girls and women throughout the extensive regions occupied by Japan where a licensed system of prostitution had already been instituted. Though the exact number cannot be estimated, in excess of two hundred thousand women and girls were "recruited"—kidnapped and coerced—into forced prostitution during the Pacific War. After the war, the survivors lived in shamed silence about their past; society was unreceptive to their stories of sexual degradation. It would be fifty years before a confluence of forces at the intersection of geopolitics, transnational feminist activism, and the memorial politics involved in fiftieth-anniversary celebrations of the end of World War II made it possible for women to bring their stories to an international arena through the auspices of the human-rights regime. In the late 1980s, women's activists within South Korea, particularly the South Korean Church Women's Alliance and the Korean Council, brought their critiques of Japanese sex tourism and the sex trade around United States military bases in Korea to national attention, emphasizing how such businesses were neoimperial forms of state-sanctioned exploitation of Korean women. The continued invocation of *wianbu* (comfort women) to refer to women in the sex trade linked earlier and contemporary forms of sexual oppression.[2]

The rights regime, and most particularly the emergent discourses of women's rights as human rights, provided the former sex prisoners a collective project (demands for apology and reparation), a social identity ("former comfort woman"), an international platform, and a story about "rape" through which the past could be newly defined. And yet, the power of the prostitution script (that these women were not forced to sexual slavery but elected the life of prostitution) enabled those unwilling to acknowledge and credit stories of sexual slavery to dismiss any claims for apology and reparation. These elderly women were asked to tell their stories of sexual degradation over and over, to activists and human-rights officials, before tribunals, and on college campuses. While the rights regime offered venues for telling their stories, however, it also had the effect of placing the women on trial. Their stories of exploitation could be negated, their legitimacy as rights claimants challenged. Moreover, the campaign on behalf of the former sex prisoners gained international momentum in the West only after the publication of Jan Ruff-O'Herne's *50 Years of Silence* in 1994. A witness to sex slavery in Dutch Indonesia, Ruff-O'Herne acknowledges that she published her narrative because the cause of the former comfort women would gain more attention if a personal testimony came from a white, Western woman.

In "Bug Chasing, Barebacking, and the Risks of Care," Gregory Tomso offers an astute and chastening analysis of the discursive tropes through which popular and scientific writing represents the "problem" of barebacking and bug chasing within the gay community in the

United States. In his meditation on the ethics of care and the problem of violence that arise with interventions in the HIV/AIDS pandemic, Tomso proposes an "ethics of the question" that challenges the explanation produced by scientists and popular writers as they confront the issue of motivation. Attentive to the "cultural unconscious of gay male sexuality at work in both scientific and popular discourses," he reveals how such writings "performatively construct bug chasing and barebacking as *moral* phenomena, since it is through the prescriptions and proscriptions of normative morality that these phenomena are named, referenced, and debated." In effect, such discourses assume behaviors to be aberrant that they produce as aberrant. Writing against the moral imperative of those who would "save" gay men from their own "self-destructive" sexual practices, Tomso refuses simplistic explanatory paradigms for "knowing" "sexual risk-takers" and calls for seeing barebacking and bug chasing "less as markers of pathological identity and more as behaviors motivated by ever-changing combinations of choices, blockages, fears, and desires that constitute both the life-affirming and life-denying practices of contemporary gay male life."

Several issues implicit in Tomso's essay interest me. One issue has to do with the value of personal witnessing. In his side argument about the uses of the popular within scientific discourse, Tomso suggests that the invocation of popular voices writing on barebacking and bug chasing offers the personal as an affective antidote to the rigidities and rationality of the putatively "scientific." He suggests that scientific writing "needs" popular writing on barebackers and bug chasers because it puts a human face on the topic and creates the truth effect of speaking from the authority of the first person. The writing of popular gay writers becomes critical—otherness is accorded authority to speak from within the experiential arena of gay male sexuality in order to bolster the authoritative claims of the scientific voice. This affective appeal of the personal voice, of first-person testimony, operates at once to sensationalize, sentimentalize, and yet paradoxically to demonize and tame the otherness of the other.

A second issue that interests me in Tomso's essay has to do with the confusion of the position of the victim that the barebacker and the bug chaser introduce into the humanitarian project of "betterment" (which itself others and subordinates the one who would be bettered). The moral indictment of the other, in this case the barebacker and the bug chaser, confuses the project of medical intervention in the sexual practices of the other. Is this other a victim to be saved? Or is this other a victimizer, a violator of someone else's, or his own, human rights? What would happen if activists working in the context of the human-rights regime, which generates new rights violations as more and more people find its efficacy enabling, organized to name the barebacker and bug chaser as perpetrators violating the sexual rights of others? Or if the barebackers and bug chasers claimed the language of rights to intervene in the social project of their betterment? What happens to this picture when the point of reference moves out of the United States to places like South Africa, where the HIV/AIDS pandemic is radically altering the social, educational, political, and economic landscape? What happens when the person practicing unprotected sex is a heterosexual man who uses virginal children as a source of uncontaminated sex? What ethics of the question arises when the differing situations of persons engaged in unprotected sex and sexual risk taking are juxtaposed?

Sexuality and dis-sexuality also figure in the act of traumatic remembering, as Lisa Diedrich explores in "'Without us all told': Paul Monette's Vigilant Witnessing to the AIDS Crisis." With Kelly Oliver's work on witnessing as her frame, Diedrich offers a compelling reading of Monette's autobiographical practice of mourning, what Nancy K. Miller and Susanna Egan term "autothanatography," the performative of narrating life at the limit of the narrator's, or another's, undoing.[3] Monette, in his "vigilant witnessing" to the HIV/AIDS crisis, attends to the other/lover and to the other in himself, representing these as the grounds of an ethics, not of recognition, but of difference and of becoming. Through Monette's work, Diedrich examines the paradox of witnessing, its absolute necessity and its impossibility. Yet this essay prompts me to consider the way in which Western literature on trauma has become the prevailing paradigm for thinking about the processes of victimization, remembering, witnessing, and recovering from the ravages and violations of the body, and how psychoanalysis has become the normative explanatory framework for approaching the complexities of the survivor's embodiment of trauma, memories of the traumatic past, and "working-through" of trauma's unpredictable disruptions in the present.

Recently, critics have vigorously debated the Western assumption of the universality of a psychoanalytic model and of the drama of "working-through." For activists and scholars working in dispersed global locations, the traumatic model, with its exclusive focus on the interiority of trauma, seems inadequate to address diverse experiential histories, languages of suffering, structures of feeling, and storytelling modes.[4] Those contesting the hegemony of the psychoanalytic model note how it privileges narratives that unfold through traumatic remembering and tell particular stories of suffering, and how it silences stories not told through the trope of trauma.[5] For such critics, the trauma model universalizes heterogeneous structures of feelings, thereby undervaluing gender, class, racial, and ethnic differences. The trauma model takes individual suffering and psychic interiority to be the ground of trauma, which obscures the modes of cultural transmission of stories and their embeddedness in political and institutional practices and structures. It also fails to address the architectures and genealogies of cultural memory or of world memory adequately. For many cultures, the trope of trauma and recovery may hold little efficacy in peoples' responses to and confrontations with a past of suffering and loss. This is all to suggest that in the midst of psychoanalysis's caution about the impossibility of testifying from the inside and the attempt to "bear witness to the inarticulate experience of the inside," we might leave open a space for thinking about other modes of witnessing and recovery.[6] Or we might attend to the ways in which particular stories of witnessing, such as Monette's, or victimization, such as that of Vietnam's "girls," are historically determined—how the stories become intelligible at specific historical moments, and how the narrator is always situated within webs of power relations that allow certain people to tell their stories while silencing others, occluding their stories of sexuality and dis-sexuality.

NOTES

1. Ronit Lentin, "The Feminisation of Catastrophe: Narrating Women's Silences," in *Global Feminist Politics: Identities in a Changing World*, ed. Suki Ali, Kelly Coate and Wangui wa Goro (New York: Routledge, 2000), 96.

2. Vera Mackie, "Sexual Violence, Silence, and Human Rights Discourse," in *Human Rights and Gender Politics: Asia-Pacific Perspectives*, ed. Anne Marie Hilsdon et al. (London: Routledge, 2000), 46.

3. Nancy K. Miller, "Representing Others: Gender and the Subjects of Autobiography," *differences: A Journal of Feminist Cultural Studies*. 6, no. 2 (1994): 1–27; and Susanna Egan, *Mirror Talk: Genres of Crisis in Contemporary Autobiography* (Chapel Hill: University of North Carolina Press, 1999).

4. See Jill Bennett and Roseanne Kennedy, *World Memory: Personal Trajectories in Global Time* (London: Palgrave, 2003).

5. See Karyn Ball, "Introduction: Trauma and Its Institutional Destinies," *Cultural Critique* 46 (Fall 2000): 1–44; Lauren Berlant, "The Subject of True Feeling: Pain, Privacy, and Politics," in *Cultural Pluralism, Identity Politics, and the Law*, ed. Austin Sarat and Thomas R. Hearns (Ann Arbor: University of Michigan Press, 1999), 49–84; and Megan Boler, "The Risks of Empathy: Interrogating Multiculturalism's Gaze," *Cultural Studies* 11, no. 2 (1997): 253–73.

6. Kelly Oliver, *Witnessing: Beyond Recognition* (Minneapolis: University of Minnesota Press, 2001), 90.

Memento Morbi: Lam Qua's Paintings, Peter Parker's Patients

Stephen Rachman

I. A Face Withheld

From the shadows of an undefined space, a room featureless in its darkness, a shrouded, semirecumbent figure reluctantly presents itself to the viewer (figure 1). The nineteenth-century Cantonese artist known to westerners as Lam Qua (Guan Qiaochang), who painted this portrait in the late 1830s, chose a restricted palette. It is a study in black, brown, and dull, mellow flesh tones. A dim source provides the bare minimum of light necessary to discern the flowing folds of the figure's dark, unstructured garment and one or two bricks (or perhaps pillows) for support. This is a medical illustration, putatively made to aid in the understanding of the patient's condition, portraying two arms (one horribly diseased, one normal) and an obstructed view of the patient's face. The distinctive visual economy of Lam Qua's composition invites the viewer to compare the arms, the normal and the pathological, but no other information, not even the sex of the patient, can be determined.[1] The patient conceals his or her face with the good hand and arm, and the fingers splay from temple to temple across its features in a timeless gesture of grief and mortification. It may take several moments for the eye to orient itself, to be sure of what one is looking at, because the diseased hand scarcely looks like a hand at all. The growth takes on a life of its own. Fungoid, disklike protuberances give it a porcine appearance as if the patient held, improbable as it must seem, a pig-faced puppet. Then in the top far-left corner, one sees the trapped thumb and fingers, dangling like a helpless claw, crowded out by the tumor, establishing the basic visual sense of the painting.

Perhaps the most extraordinary of a remarkable series of at least 114 paintings made between 1836 and 1852 in Lam Qua's studio, it depicts one of the Chinese patients of a leading medical missionary, Rev. Dr. Peter Parker, an American Presbyterian minister and physician.[2] In late 1835, Parker opened the Ophthalmic Hospital in Canton (Guangzhou). He soon acquired a reputation as a surgeon of such skill that his eye infirmary became a general hospital in which he treated thousands of cases. Arguing that medicine could be the "handmaid of religious truth," he offered free medical care as a way to bring the Chinese to God and held regular services in the hospital.[3] Among the thousands of patients were a number afflicted with mature tumors (as much as thirty-five years old), which Parker had Lam Qua, who was trained in both Western and Chinese styles of painting and maintained a busy studio very close to Parker's hospital, paint in the days before photography.[4] When viewed in the context of Parker's corresponding case notes, Lam Qua's paintings become even more complex images of cultural confluence and exchange, of East and West, Orient and Occident, portraiture and clinical documentation, Christian and heathen, rich and poor.

In this essay, I will address the ways in which the clinical and aesthetic values of Lam Qua's paintings are intimately bound up in that confluence, in the fragmented histories of patients, a cross-cultural collaboration between a doctor and a painter, and a period of momentous political and medical change. Analysis of these images, when linked to Parker's case histories, reveals the collaboration and contestation of the Chinese and the American at a moment when notions of these terms were in embryonic stages of development.

Lam Qua's portrait of a patient concealing her face stands as a rarity in the history of nineteenth-century painting and in the annals of medical representation. The conventions of modern clinical representation preserve anonymity by cropping the face or blacking out the eyes; here the patient obscures identity by withholding the gaze, the visage. Despite celebrated examples such as Rembrandt's *Dr. Tulp's Anatomy Lesson* and Thomas Eakins's monumental portraits of the clinicians Samuel Gross and D. Hayes Agnew, oil paintings—with the exception of doctors' portraits—of medical subjects are relatively rare, and portraits of patients with tumors of such size and deformity rarer still. When not employing photography, most medical illustration was and continues to be drawn. It categorizes by taxonomy and specimen. Western nineteenth-century images of the abject subjected to the gaze of science and made to sit for clinical purposes seldom reveal the sitter's prerogative to hide from the artist, doctor, or lens of the recording instrument, from what Foucault might have called the eye of power.[5] In nineteenth-century scientific images of the criminal, diseased, mad, or enslaved, the objects of study do not withhold them-

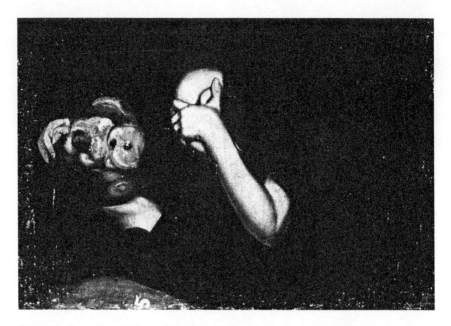

FIGURE 1. Lam Qua, *Patient of Dr. Peter Parker (Leäng Yen)*, circa 1838. Oil on canvas, 24 x 18 in. Reproduced by permission of Yale University, Harvey Cushing/John Hay Whitney Medical Library (no. 5 in Peter Parker Collection).

selves. The faces that appear in Rogue's Galleries, Hugh Welch Diamond's photographs of the insane, J. T. Zealy's daguerreotypes of slaves, medical-record photographs of the gunshot wounds of Civil War soldiers, and even Jean-Martin Charcot's hysterics are all presented as more or less acquiescent objects of scientific attention.[6]

But the figure in Lam Qua's painting will not or cannot sit openly or stoically for this portrait. Rather, we see a starkly emotional drama in which the good hand performs an act of concealment while the bad hand is held up for all to see. The suffering is rendered anonymous and becomes emblematic of the raw, direct trauma of illness and the hidden quality of individual suffering despite the attempts of medicine to disclose it. The patient cannot confront what we can scarcely look at ourselves and, therefore, the significance of the image is suspended in a grotesque of beholding and withholding. The "grotesque," a term derived from the strange images found in Roman caves or "grottoes," has been conventionally understood as an incongruous or unnatural combination of the human, animal, or monstrous that provokes incongruous or contradictory emotional reactions (e.g., fear and laughter). In *Rabelais and His World*, Mikhail Bakhtin described a comprehensive notion of "grotesque realism" that not only elicits those reactions in response to descriptions of the body and bodily functions but partakes of an infinite range of positive and negative earthly combinations, invoking both degradation and regeneration. In its distortion of the body, capacity for unregulated growth, and status as alien, yet connected tissue, a large tumor like the one visible in this painting visually confirms the ways in which growth, transformation, and the conjugation of many forms of bodily states produce the grotesque. But these paintings do not merely depict grotesque subject matter. They embody a cultural grotesque particular to Canton in the era they were produced.[7]

II. Exchange and Circulation in Canton:
Cultural Production of the Grotesque

When examined together, a striking complementarity appears in the careers of Parker and Lam Qua. Both were born in the early years of the nineteenth century and rose from relatively obscure origins to notoriety in both the East and the West. Parker was the first American medical missionary to gain wide cultural acceptance and respect for Western medicine and, to a lesser extent, Western religion in Canton; Lam Qua was the first Chinese portrait painter to be favorably exhibited in the West. Neither Parker nor Lam Qua was the first to ply his skills in his respective field, but both were much more effective than their predecessors at garnering publicity for their efforts. The acceleration of trade, trade hostilities, and print media in the 1830s and '40s allowed for much wider acclaim than was previously possible and consequently both were widely viewed in their day as pioneers who broke through longstanding cultural barriers. To some observers, neither Lam Qua nor Parker was the physical type normally associated with each chosen profession. Lam Qua's rotundity was not in keeping with stereotypical assumptions about lean and sensitive painters. Parker's large hands, coarsened by farm work, seemed indelicate for a gentleman surgeon, and casual observers were frequently surprised by their dexterity.[8] Parker took an evident interest in painting, and Lam Qua was reported to have been "a great lover of the medical profession, and regrets that he is too old to become a doctor himself."[9]

Perhaps more interestingly, Parker and Lam Qua traveled in similar social and political orbits. Of course, they had a number of direct personal connections, but they seemed to share a wide and overlapping circle of acquaintances. Lam Qua produced a number of portraits of Howqua, a powerful merchant who instrumentally provided a commercial space for Parker's hospital at 3 Hog Lane. Accounts and memoirs of Western visitors who had dealings with Lam Qua and which provide the most detailed accounts of him invariably mention Parker. No doubt this had everything to do with the claustrophobic environment of the foreign factory sector of Canton, adjacent to the old walled city. For the bulk of their acquaintance, both Parker and Lam Qua labored in this factory district, a settlement small enough to be measured in footsteps by its pent-up foreign occupants: two hundred and seventy paces from one end to the other along the riverfront and a mere fifty from the shore to the shops and factories, or hongs, as they were called. Their workplaces became favored destinations, sites of brisk traffic and frequent visits. Not only did they live and work in or adjacent to factories, they both came to oversee factories, as it were (Parker in his hospital treating one hundred patients a day, Lam Qua in his studio), using the methods of manufacturing and employing teams of assistants to handle the demand for their services. Both were well connected among their own countrymen, but, ultimately, it was their mutual ability to attract friends and admirers among foreign populations that drew them together.

By 1835, when Parker opened the Ophthalmic Hospital in Canton (originally he intended to specialize in eye disease), Lam Qua was already the city's preeminent export painter.[10] According to slightly varied accounts by foreign visitors, his studio on New China Street advertised, in the midst of Chinese characters, "Lam-qua, English and Chinese Painter," or "Handsome-face Painter." He sold portraits to a mixed clientele in the "English fashion" or, at a 20 percent discount, in the "China fashion."[11] He was thought to be "a great portrait painter among the Chinese" and the finest Chinese painter by westerners.[12] His paintings were exhibited at the Royal Academy in London and in France, New York, Boston, and Philadelphia.[13] In the late 1860s, the English photographer John Thomson, who was undertaking his well-known study of China, wrote admiringly of Lam Qua, "Lumqua [*sic*] produced a number of excellent works in oil, which are still copied by the painters in Hong Kong and Canton. Had he lived in any other country he would have been the founder of a school of painting."[14]

Though the details are contradictory, Lam Qua had been influenced by a distinguished English painter of the China coast, George

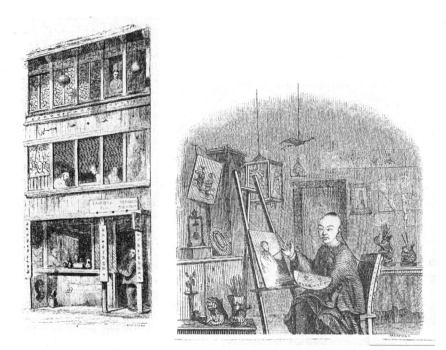

FIGURES 2 & 3. Reprinted from Paul Emile Daurand Forgues [Old Nick, pseud.], *La Chine Ouverte* (Paris: H. Fournier, 1845), 56. Exterior and interior of Lam Qua's studio. Figure 3 is supposed to be Lam Qua himself although Lam Qua reportedly painted standing up. Here we are meant to see the amalgam of Chinese and European techniques as he sits with Western palette and easel but holds the brush in the Chinese manner.

Chinnery, who arrived in Macao in the mid-1820s with a more flamboyant mode of portraiture.[15] Lam Qua soon assimilated Chinnery's style into his own. Eventually the two had a falling out, probably due to the fact the Lam Qua could undercut Chinnery's business by offering, as Patrick Conner has explained, "the novelty of an accomplished work in the Western style by a Chinese artist—and at a fraction of the price."[16] It is not surprising to find friction in these relations and not just for business reasons; the subtlety and distinction of Western fine arts traditions were a matter of considerable cultural pride and bias. On the one hand, westerners like Chinnery obviously wished to expose the Chinese to European art forms and influence them; on the other hand, these skills were perceived as a mark of cultural superiority. A French critic, de la Vollée, suggested that Lam Qua was "out of his element before an [*sic*] European countenance" and liable to *"China-fy"* Anglo-American faces (albeit with inadvertent originality).[17]

But the rise of Lam Qua and several other artists as genuinely accomplished masters of English portraiture indicated otherwise—these qualities were indeed transferable—and signaled an intensification of cultural and commercial competition that marked the second half of the 1830s and the period of the opium wars. In fact, the way Lam Qua wedded the mass production of images to the production of unique likenesses of Western faces astonished visitors. Typically, Western observers in Canton were deeply preoccupied with comparing Chinese and Western technology, knowledge, and modes of production. They were especially sensitive to the spectacle of Chinese artisans cranking out conventional landscapes for the Western market. Describing this part of Lam Qua's workshop, a French observer wrote, "There is no art in this. It is purely a mechanical operation." This line of thought quickly extended to all of Chinese culture.[18] Through the lens of cultural condescension, the modernity of the "picture business" in Canton was (mis)understood by many Western visitors as another sign of Chinese backwardness. The desire for reassurance of the superiority of Western artistry and the mentality that produced it easily obscured the flexibility and assimilative power of Lam Qua's art operations. Western visitors continually sought to memorialize themselves in oil, to bring back souvenirs of Canton and the Chinese, and Lam Qua accommodated all of these demands with a surprisingly modern mixture of mass production and personal artistry. His studio was, in a manner of speaking, another kind of grotesque, tailored to the nineteenth-century Occidental mentality, combining factory models of production with the romantic notion of the autonomous individual artist.

Commerce in Canton also produced a linguistic grotesquerie fundamental to the work of Parker and Lam Qua. Because of the scarcity of translators or multilingual speakers, all who did business there resorted to a pidgin language (pidgin derives from a Cantonese pronunciation of business or "pidginess"). Rooted in Chinese syntax and phraseology and absorbing words from Portuguese and Indian as well as English and Chinese dialects, this commercial patter had to be picked up on the fly by Western speakers. Cantonese businesses kept handwritten phrase books of the jargon and it was "deemed one of the first steps to the acquisition of English, to copy out one of these manuscripts."[19] Non-English speakers were frequently confounded. English speakers felt simultaneously amused and degraded by having to listen to and speak this pidgin language and saw it as another sign of Chinese resistance and hostility.[20] If the grotesque, as I have suggested above, provokes alienation via incongruous or contradictory reactions such as fear and laughter, then Canton elicited this response in foreign visitors linguistically via Pidgin English. The proliferation in the 1830s and '40s of the translation of the Chinese *yi* as "barbarian" and the surprising number of Western memoirs in which visitors refer to themselves by the epithet *Fan–Kwae* or *Fan-Qui*, or "foreign devils," indicate to some extent the degree to which westerners registered their alienation.[21]

Peter Parker established the Ophthalmic Hospital in the midst of this commercial and linguistic hotbed. He believed that the hospital could genuinely facilitate "social and friendly intercourse" between Chinese and foreigners, diffuse knowledge of Euro-American arts and sciences, and, above all, replace "pitiable superstitions" with the gospel truth. As he saw it, the key to reaching the "millions of this partially civilized yet *'mysterious'* and idolatrous empire" was that his work must be entirely without fee, free from any form of "pecuniary remuneration." At all times, his motive "must appear to be one of *disinterested benevolence.*"[22] A sign was placed over the entrance to the hospital that read *P'u Ai I Yuan* (Hospital of Universal Love).

In a city utterly dedicated to getting and spending, gratuitous care raised suspicion among the hong merchants. They assumed that Parker must have some ulterior motive and placed him under surveillance, planting a spy (who worked as a linguist) in the hospital.[23] Of course, his motive was to gain influence and converts, but there was nothing particularly devious about it. In 1836, Parker declared, "We cannot suppose the fond parent will remain insensible to the obligations of gratitude when he returns to his home, or fail to speak there of the *excluded foreigner* who had gratuitously restored his child to the blessings of health. We conceive there cannot be a more direct avenue to influence than will be presented in this department."[24]

In 1872, nearing the end of his career, Parker assessed his success. He reflected on his work at the hospital, but he remembered as well his part in negotiating the United States' first treaty with China in the mid-1840s. He claimed that during one of the negotiations over the lease of land for building sites in the treaty ports, a Chinese deputy minister "whose father and mother had been my patients" suggested that "temples of worship" be included in the list. Parker had removed polyps from the nose of the father, and he believed that the son's deep gratitude had inspired him to permit Western churches in China. Surgical success thus served as the "entering wedge" in the treaty and promised to make possible the evangelization of China. Parker asserted that the minister offered this provision "knowing the gratification it would afford me."[25] Such was Parker's faith in the power of filial gratitude and his medical mission. In Parker's theory, gratitude for bodies cured was a path to the Chinese souls he wished to save.

In practice, the hospital gave Parker unprecedented access to the Chinese body of all ages and classes, male and female, from near and far. Originally, Parker intended to treat primarily eye diseases such as blindness (which was reportedly very widespread) and secondarily, the deaf and dumb; one hears the aura of Christ at Bethesda in this decision: to make the blind see, the deaf hear, the mute speak. An early case note from November 1835 reveals Parker ministering to Akeen, a thirty-one-year-old blind merchant, telling him (through an interpreter) "of the world in which he may see, though never again on earth; that in heaven none are blind, none deaf, none sick."[26] One might wonder in just what way Parker's *joss pidgin* (religious service) was lost in translation, but while Parker was urging admittance to the celestial infirmary, hundreds of Chinese were lining up for admittance to his earthly one. In his first year, he received over two thousand and one hundred patients with cataracts and a host of eye complaints, tumors, abscesses, cancer, goiters, bladder stones, scoliosis, hepatitis, pneumonia, impetigo, ulcers, and "opium mania." Each day, patients would line up by the hundreds, a porter would issue them numbered bamboo tickets, and the doctor would see as many as he could. The ferocious demand for his services could scarcely be met and like a line worker coping with a ruthless speedup, Parker worked himself into a state of exhaustion.

Nor would the gratitude he inspired always come in what he deemed theologically acceptable forms. Grateful patients frequently kowtowed to him and he was at pains to pull them from the floor; one patient even requested a painting of Parker to which he might offer daily prayers. But the cases came before him in an endless, inundating stream, compelling him to revise his medical/spiritual agenda. The encounters were intense and complex and it was the pressure of this onslaught that inspired Parker's collaboration with Lam Qua. Exactly why Parker requested that Lam Qua paint these portraits is not entirely clear.[27] Lam Qua was the uncle of Kwan A-to, Parker's first Chinese pupil in Western surgery, and it has been remarked that the paintings were made as tokens of gratitude for Parker's effort and skill, which he plied without remuneration. Lam Qua is reported to have said "that as there is no charge for 'cutting,' [pidgin for surgery] he can make none for painting."[28] This reciprocity, however, is complicated by the fact that

Parker's ledgers for 1851 show that twenty-five dollars were paid for "Lamqua [sic] paintings of tumors."[29]

The enormous size of the tumors and the surgical challenges they presented warranted illustration. They simply had to be seen to be believed. Parker probably planned to donate them to the Anatomical Museum of the Medical Missionary Society in China, a group formed in the late 1830s to institutionalize the medical-missionary approach exemplified by Parker and his English and American colleagues, but that museum never came about.[30] He did, however, deposit a set of portraits at Guy's Hospital in London, which may have been an expression of the original plan.[31] Upon his return to the United States in 1840–1, Parker used the paintings on at least one occasion to illustrate his lectures before medical audiences as a way to advertise his work, raise funds for the hospital, and recruit young missionary doctors.[32]

The paintings functioned for Parker as visual testimonials to his medical skill and to the nature of the Chinese as he found them. He selected patients to be painted on a principle similar to the one he used to cull the cases worth reporting from the thousands that came through the hospital doors. Some cases were chosen, as he wrote in 1848, "for their interest in a surgical point of view, others illustrating different shades of the character of the Chinese."[33] Like the many scrolls of tribute that grateful Chinese patients would frequently bestow on Parker, the paintings emphasized the magnitude of the task he had accomplished.[34] In a portrait commemorating Parker's work at the hospital and his instruction of Kwan A-to, Lam Qua bestowed upon Parker his own scroll as it were, painting it on the wall behind the doctor (figure 4). The paintings may have served as visual proof of the necessity of devoting the majority of his time to medical care instead of evangelizing. Parker's relations with his religious sponsors, the American Board of Commissioners for Foreign Missions, grew tense because of the board's concern that Parker was spending too much time healing bodies; by 1847 the board would sever its connections with Parker over this issue.[35] The paintings must have served as a form of spiritual compensation for the doctor who took no fees, a way of taking and maintaining possession of his patients. "God has signally smiled upon efforts to benefit the body," Parker noted in his journal for March 1843. "It was from the bended knee in one room that I went to take the knife in another. God heard the petition offered."[36]

From chapel to table, from prayer to cutting, the doctor moved, and he saw surgical outcomes (at least the positive ones) in providential terms. Many of the paintings were, indirectly, the mementos of an-

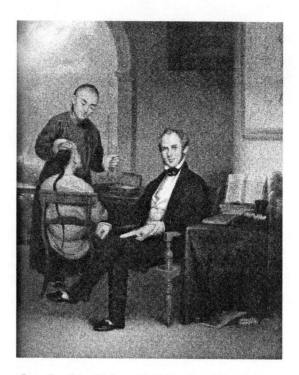

FIGURE 4. Lam Qua, *Dr. Peter Parker with his Student Kwan A-to*, circa 1840s. Oil on canvas, 25.5 x 20.5 in. Courtesy of Peter Parker V. The scroll in the upper-right corner is addressed to Dr. Parker, who "through the magic of his hands, restores youthful health, and gives longevity and life for the benefit of the people." The high commissioner Kíying bestowed this scroll.

swered prayers, visual analogues for his entire missionary enterprise. Grotesque fusings of diseased bodies and the strivings of a missionary doctor, Lam Qua's paintings become, as my title is intended to suggest, *memento morbi*, tokens of disease and cure.

III. Likeness and Representation

How then is the cultural grotesque manifested in Lam Qua's paintings of Parker's patients? Sander Gilman argues:

In Lam Qua's paintings the patient becomes an extension of the pathology . . . much as the English country gentlemen in [Sir

Thomas] Lawrence's paintings become representative of a class or an attitude toward life. In Lam Qua's paintings the patient "vanishes" since the patient becomes the perceived object shared between the physician-missionary, Peter Parker, who is lecturing about them, and his Western audience. . . . The patient bears a double stigma—first, the sign of pathology, and second, the sign of barbarism, his Chinese identity.[37]

But this view unnecessarily conflates Lam Qua's paintings with their presumed Western reception, suggesting that because a Chinese artist paints in a Western mode, the meaning of painting and all of its effects are wholly subsumed under that system. It suggests that under the discursive field of Western science, Parker's patients become little more than their diseases and evidence of the Chinese heathen. While it is certainly true that paintings did function in a missionary discourse that trafficked in notions of cultural superiority and inferiority, I propose that we consider these paintings in terms that more accurately account for their resonance and power.

"I am indebted to Lam Qua," Parker explained in his case notes on Lew Akin, a young girl on whom he operated in April 1837, "who has taken an admirable likeness of the little girl and a good representation of the tumor."[38] Lam Qua's paintings achieve their complexity and power, in part, because of the duality to which Parker alludes. These images are indeed at once likenesses and representations. In the best examples, the sensitivity with which the admirable likeness of an individual is delineated contrasts against the details of the true representation of the tumors. Parker's distinction is an interesting one. In all probability, he uses *likeness* in the old, conventional sense as a term of resemblance appropriate to portraiture (of persons), and *representation* as a term of resemblance appropriate to objects, a usage connoting graphic realism—likeness for people, representation for things. But it is also a distinction that is useful to help understand the power of these images and how medical imaging functions.

The difference between likeness and representation signifies not so much different modes of painting per se as it does different ways of seeing. The likeness is the visual category in which one seeks to recognize the particularity of an individual: features, symmetry, marks of identification. For Parker, these images of former patients (*memento morbi*) whom he could recognize by sight must have retained a personal value and served as a memory aid. Also, he had personal knowledge of the fidelity of any given likeness that Lam Qua produced. But because these individuals are unknown to us, their likeness functions on a different level of identification—a way of seeing the broader categories of the normative human, the male or female, the old or young, beautiful or plain, or perhaps the ethnic/racial category of the Chinese.[39] We also attend to the aspect of the face and eyes for any expressive or affective signs.

The representation functions as a visual category in which one observes objects by type or classification, be it medical or some other system. It stands for some part of the body or some kind of growth, the pathological or non-normative. Lam Qua's images frequently invoke in the viewer a kind of gestalt where the eye and the mind travel between the likeness and the representation, the normal and the pathological, the subject and the object. For this reason, I suggest, the tumor often appears as the patient's prop, as a musician might pose with his cello, while the eye of the beholder shuttles between these two ways of seeing.[40] In the case of Woo Kinshing, "aged 49, a fisherman from Shihszetow, near the Bogue," a ten-year-old tumor had "attained a very great magnitude resembling in figure a tenor viol." Because the shape and size of Woo Kinshing's tumor resembles a familiar object, a cello or "tenor viol" as Parker calls it, Lam Qua's image raises another issue of pathological representation latent in many images (figure 5). What happens to the status of the tumor when it resembles an ordinary nonpathological object? In Woo Kinshing's case, the suggestion of the cello is reinforced by the coincidence of it being positioned more or less where a cellist might play it. The tumor becomes a prop; in fact, Woo Kinshing would rest on it like a mattress. The indirection or redirection of the pathological gaze toward some other object frequently produces a ludicrous effect, and a kind of "tumor humor" emerges. Referring to the tumor as the patient's "old companion" and calling Woo Kinshing at several points "the old gentleman" (though he was only forty-nine), a lighter tone enters Parker's case history, especially given how difficult the surgery proved to be.[41]

In the case of Kwan Meiurh, we see a middle-aged woman, "a silk embroiderer," with "a preternatural development of the left mamma" (figure 6). Parker reported that a Chinese physician "applied to it a succession of plasters. Soon after the integument ulcerated and the gland protruded." The woman was in agony. Parker reported that "she was much emaciated and the breast, one third as large as her head, came down as low as the umbilicus." The dignified stoicism of Kwan Meiurh's portrait is consistent with Parker's account of the case. Though the operation was without anesthetic, the patient hardly made a sound.

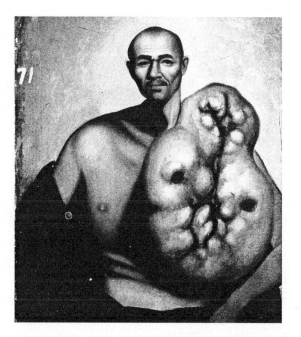

FIGURE 5. Lam Qua, *Patient of Dr. Peter Parker (Woo Kinshing)*, circa 1838. Oil on canvas, 24 x 18 in. Reproduced by permission of Yale University, Harvey Cushing/ John Hay Whitney Medical Library (no. 71 in Peter Parker Collection).

"The composed and confiding manner in which she came to the operation," he observed, "could not escape the notice of the gentlemen who were present. Apparently no child ever lay in the arms of its parent with more confidence of safety, than this woman lay upon the operation table under the knife of a foreigner."[42] Parker's obvious admiration for the patient extended beyond her high tolerance for pain (a characteristic of Chinese patients that continually inspired awe in Parker and his colleagues). He was pleased with her matter-of-fact attitude toward the necessity of the operation, her sense of the relative pain of surgery vis-à-vis the disease, and her, according to his account, childlike trust in his surgical power. Lam Qua appears to have brilliantly captured Kwan Meiurh's stately strength in the tension between the face and the growth, a comparison invited by the comment about the growth's size with respect to the patient's head. While Parker's paternalism is fully on display (he seems to veritably revel in her confidence in him), it also elicits an expression of his own distance from

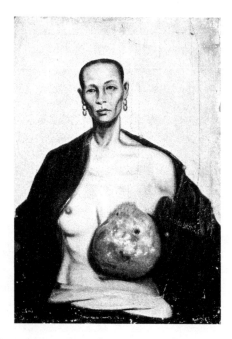

FIGURE 6. Lam Qua, *Patient of Dr. Peter Parker (Kwan Meiurh)*, circa 1838. Oil on canvas, 24 x 18 in. Reproduced by permission of Yale University, Harvey Cushing/ John Hay Whitney Medical Library (no. 29 in Peter Parker Collection).

her as a surgeon and an outsider. She is almost too confident, too trusting "under the knife of a foreigner." Parker's sense of the patient's "deliverance" is the only hint of religiosity in the account. He directs his real animus against what he perceived as the quackery and mal-treatment that the patient suffered at the hands of traditional Chinese practitioners. In complex ways, therefore, the grotesque is organized and reorganized by the case histories and the images, producing powerful and contradictory effects by shuttling between these two modalities.

IV. Leäng Yen

Let us return to the image of the withheld face of the Chinese patient, this time supplying a case history that corresponds to it. The person in this painting matches Parker's description of Leäng Yen, a thirty-four-year-old woman from the neighborhood of Hwate, who first visited the Canton Hospital in the fall of 1838.[43] During the previous October, she stopped menstruating and noticed a swelling in her right arm near the wrist. It had been neither remarkably painful nor especially bloody, but it had grown very rapidly. By the time she ventured to the hospital it was the size of a log measuring nineteen inches in circumference. Parker observed that her complexion had taken on a sickly pale-yellow hue. Fluid had built up, the swelling was considerable in her right arm, and her pulse was weak and fast. Her appetite was good; too good, in fact, for the doctor thought it was "morbid," driven by her condition. He admitted her as his 5,721st case (in just under three years), put her on blue pill (a mercury-based compound commonly given for hypochondria, depression, constipation, etc.), colocynth (a purgative), and a few grains of opium at night to help her sleep.

Parker believed that she had an osteo-medullary sarcoma, a cancerous growth that appeared to originate in the bone and bone marrow. He felt sure he would have to amputate as soon as possible, but he had never performed an amputation on a Chinese woman before. As with all his serious cases, he consulted his English and American colleagues, most likely Dr. R. H. Cox and William Jardine, the latter being a former ship's surgeon and leading partner in the prominent English trading firm Jardine Matheson. Dr. Guilbert, of the French frigate L'Artemise, happened to be in port, and he too was consulted. The doctors stood by the patient discussing her case in English so she would not understand, but one of them made some gesture, perhaps a cutting motion, and Leäng Yen surmised what the doctors proposed. She was completely against it. But unable to confront the medical men directly, she told someone else that "she would sooner die than submit to the operation" (576). The doctors explained to her that they felt that she badly needed the operation, that it "would not be extremely painful" (this occurred before the introduction of anesthesia), and that she would soon die without it (577). Leäng Yen replied that she would be utterly helpless without her right hand. She conceded that it was better to lose a limb than the whole body, but she still felt at odds with the procedure. After a few days, she left the hospital and went home.

About three weeks later she returned to the hospital with her husband. She seemed to be in better health—Parker attributed this to the medication he had placed her on—but the tumor had grown even larger with fungoid protrusions. Once again the doctors proposed to amputate, and this time both she and her husband consented. However, since this was such an extraordinary undertaking, Leäng Yen's husband felt that he had best consult with his wife's family. He returned home and found that the family approved of the doctor's recommendation, but he then fell sick and could not travel. He wrote to Parker, giving his unqualified consent. When Leäng Yen learned that her husband would not be with her for the operation, she grew anxious. She was afraid that if he were not present and something went wrong, preventing her full recovery, he "might decline to support her" (577). She was assured that "if he deserted her, she should be provided for," and the operation was scheduled for December 5, 1838 (577). All was in readiness on that morning, but when the doctor met with his patient he learned that she had changed her mind again. According to Parker, "with a toss of her head" she shouted, 'No cutting! No cutting!' and holding up two fingers she added, 'Give 200 dollars and you may'" (577).

Thwarted and disconcerted by the complete breakdown in communication between doctor and patient—especially Leäng Yen's sense of the doctor's motives—Parker endeavored to explain that he was not "anxious to mutilate her" and that he would not "give her price to do it" (577). He wondered how she could fail to realize that she had been provided food and a female servant to attend to her every need for her own benefit. Parker felt that, in her refusal, she was an "exception to all that have ever yet visited the hospital" (577). In the face of this, Leäng Yen backed away from her demand, saying that someone else had suggested to her that the two hundred dollars "would make her independent of her husband for support" (577). Parker wrote to the husband of these difficulties, and in a few days, despite his illness, the husband returned to the hospital and apologized on behalf of his wife, explaining "that it was not the Chinese custom to expect the physician to pay for healing his patient" (577). Leäng Yen also "seemed ashamed for her ingratitude" (577). All parties were at last whole-heartedly agreed that the amputation was desirable.

Once more, Parker obtained from his patient the "usual indemnity" that he would not be liable if the patient should die. He felt this was all the more necessary because Leäng Yen had grown feeble during these protracted negotiations. Her pulse was alarmingly high because the tumor was exerting great vascular pressure. The operation was slated for Wednesday, December 12. Two days prior, a doctor visited the patient and expressed the opinion that "she would not live to see the day," and that she was "just able to be lifted from the bed to the table" (577). Parker's case notes record that "an opiate was administered half an hour before the time of the operation, also five grains of blue pill, and ten of ext. of rhubarb" (578). The arm was removed above the elbow. Leäng Yen, once determined to go through with the procedure, was openly contemptuous of the pain involved: "At the moment of sawing the bone [she] inquired when that part of the process would take place" (578). The operation was a success and Parker noted another ironic detail: the operation had been performed in his quiet hospital "during the time of the attempted execution of an opium dealer, and the consequent riot, in front of the factories" (578).

Examination of the removed forearm revealed disease in the marrow of the radius and ulna. Parker found the tumor to be generally surrounded by a bony plate composed of "a mass of matter the consistency of brain"(578). This substance had protruded through holes in the plate and "expanded itself like a mushroom" (578). Leäng Yen's condition stabilized after the amputation. The wound healed without infection and her only bodily difficulties appeared to be digestive. Five days after the operation, Parker discovered her devouring an oily bowl of sausages "even without rice" (578). When Parker scolded her, she "was much displeased and quite lost her temper" (578). By January 10, 1839, she was well enough to return home, but "she preferred remaining still longer where everything was provided for her" (578). Nine days later her husband returned to the hospital to collect her and she "was discharged in excellent spirits" with the prospect of life and health (578). "The opportunity," Parker concludes, "was improved in impressing upon them their obligations to the living God, and author of all their mercies" (579).

At some point in the preoperative part of her stay at the hospital, Parker most likely had Lam Qua paint Leäng Yen. The tumor described in the case notes closely resembles this image, especially with its mushroomlike protrusions and the swelling on the right side of the body (note the differences in the two arms). The feebleness of the patient and the shame Parker records her feeling in the negotiations over the operation supply a plausible context for the pose Lam Qua chose to paint (or perhaps, in which the patient consented to be painted), altering the painting's potential significance—what it was possibly intended to memorialize and the range of meanings we might ascribe to it. Reading the image anonymously, Larissa N. Heinrich suggests that "by concealing the identity of the patient, the painting still conveys a strong message about the curability of Chinese culture. . . . [T]he true nature of Chinese identity, the painting seems to say, is merely waiting for the art of Parker's scalpel to describe."[44] Once identified, the image no longer addresses the generic issues of healing, cure, and identity. Amputation, after all, would hardly restore the right hand to perfection and would certainly not yield any final revelations about Leäng Yen's identity as Chinese. Rather, the painting portrays a patient withholding herself and resisting the system of exchange that undergirds Parker's hospital mission on almost every level. We recognize the empathy of Lam Qua's artistry, which is strikingly different in tone than the vexed superciliousness of Parker's report.

Leäng Yen does not withhold her identity precisely (for the tumor still allows for identification, and Parker would presumably know the patient in question); rather she withholds her gaze, her likeness, while proffering her representation. Though she is, according to Parker, "the first Chinese female . . . at least in modern times to submit to amputation of her right arm," she will not present herself directly to Lam Qua's canvas as a subject of medical scrutiny.[45] Even as Parker relates it from his viewpoint, the case is riddled with incidents of mutual misunderstanding and tension. The patient surmises the diagnosis and treatment across the barrier of language and over and against the attempts of the medical men to conceal it. The life-saving nature of the operation is construed by the patient as a commercial or mercenary enterprise—like almost all other foreign operations in Canton. While it is unclear in which language these exchanges took place, the grotesque comedy emerges in Pidgin English with Leäng Yen shouting "No cutting!" and bargaining for the arm. Suddenly, the saintly doctor is misconstrued as a ghoul, a body-snatching anatomizer—oddly evocative of contemporaneous fears of modern medicine expressed in Western countries—and his Hospital of Universal Love from which all remuneration was to be banished is taken for a place of haggling and barter just like any other Canton hong.[46]

Parker is convinced that his patient is gaming the system of the hospital, maximizing her stay. Leäng Yen feels trapped and at risk of spousal abandonment. Caught out in her attempt to obtain financial independence by selling herself for what she perceived of as medical experimentation and then ashamed at the appearance of her own ingratitude, she is cornered by her husband into an operation she dreads. A hungry, noncompliant patient, she eats with gusto "oily sausages." With an uncanny, almost novelistic sense of setting, the operation takes place in the midst of one of the early Canton riots that touched off the opium wars—a struggle that emblematized the chaos, coercion, and rancor of Chinese and Western relations. In the language of his case notes, Parker tries to distinguish the quiet of his surgical theater from the turmoil of the streets, suggesting that his model of foreign relations is superior.

But the conflict between Leäng Yen and himself suggests that the distinction—while well-taken in general—cannot be so neatly drawn. In cultural terms, this painting is inevitably about the Chinese-Western relations that Peter Parker forged in the 1830s and '40s, mediated through the diseased body of a woman who felt trapped in a patriarchal society and was desperately in need of an operation that could only be performed by a well-meaning but equally patriarchal doctor. In the context of the case, it is this grotesque matrix of deeply human despair captured at a profound moment of crisis that Lam Qua's image conveys.

V. Memento Morbi

In both Lam Qua's portrait and in Parker's case notes, Leäng Yen occupies several middle grounds that are in many ways emblematic of differentials encompassed by what I am calling *memento morbi*. A woman in the masculine world of the factory district of Canton, she was captured between revealing and withholding, charity and commerce, and diagnosis and operation. Parker, too, occupied his own middle ground between the material and the spiritual, body and soul, and disease and health, as it were. And Lam Qua, as well, occupied a middle ground. He was a Chinese artist, as Michael Sullivan remarked of his landscapes, who by adopting "a Western technique, . . . also adopts a Western vision," a vision not quite possible through the generalized techniques of Chinese styles.[47] In the grotesque and human tension between likeness and representation, he portrayed the Chinese through Western ways of seeing.

As the use of Cantonese Pidgin English by Lam Qua, Parker, and his patients was inevitably susceptible to linguistic distortion, so the triangle of patient, doctor, and artist that is partially revealed in these paintings was fraught with the misconstrued meanings of cross-cultural negotiation. For the sitters, these paintings signify an additional encumbrance: the burden of one's mortality, growing from the side of one's face, hand, or chest, recorded for the glum significance of medical history. It is a representational process by which one becomes part of a doctor's collection. But in the instance of Leäng Yen's portrait, the anonymity of human suffering becomes something else. In the splayed hand that covers the face, we see the burden of the representation of disease expressed as a refusal to yield her likeness. And a final detail of Lam Qua's portrait emerges as we faintly discern Leäng Yen's eye, perhaps peeking out from behind that hand; the likeness, as it were, not wholly blinding itself to the very process it resists.

As the significance of these portraits sits at the busy intersection of medicine, history, and culture, they also traffic in meanings circumscribed by artistic practices. Oil painting on canvas is in general a laborious, time-consuming process. In generic terms, portraiture often entails multiple sittings and perhaps sketches and studies in a formal, frequently monumentalizing set of procedures. Despite Lam Qua's obvious skill, the medium was not well suited to capturing the radical transformations of Parker's surgery and the cellular minutia of gross pathology. Lam Qua's studio, with its divisions of labor, was undoubtedly capable of quickly producing images, but this meant that the images had to be of necessity stereotypical.[48] While oil on canvas was perhaps the best that early nineteenth-century technology had to offer, it is important to keep in mind that, if the paintings were to be used primarily in a pathological museum, then the typical midrange viewpoint they provide could be improved upon. But what is lost in close-up medical scrutiny is gained in the tension of likeness and representation inherent in these paintings. Lam Qua's portraits of Parker's patients are anything but stereotypical; they capture patients in relation to their condition in a moment of preoperative stasis, or, as in the case of Leäng Yen, crisis. We are compelled to value Lam Qua's portraits for the way a painstaking medium is made to yield to the urgency of disease and the fears of impending surgery and possible death.

Similarly, the pressure for beds in Parker's hospital mandated that postoperative convalescence should take no longer than necessary. (This would be the administrative rationale for Parker's irritation at Leäng Yen's tarrying during her recovery.) It is likely that for these reasons Lam Qua only produced one before-and-after sequence for Parker, that of the laborer Po Ashing who had his left arm amputated at the Canton Hospital in 1838 (figures 7 and 8). When time or circumstance permitted, Lam Qua produced portraits of patients with the accoutrements of the studio, as in the case of Po Ashing's postoperative portrait—he is posed in a landscape. But other images, like Leäng Yen's and some hastily rendered portraits were obviously composed with greater speed and in less artistically favorable conditions (probably at the hospital). In this way, the artistry of Lam Qua emerges under medical pressure. Parker and Lam Qua shared a common burden of serving the masses that would daily stream through hospital and studio one at a time. Cutting and painting find their ultimate equivalency in these images and in the lives and cases of the individuals they represent. Like

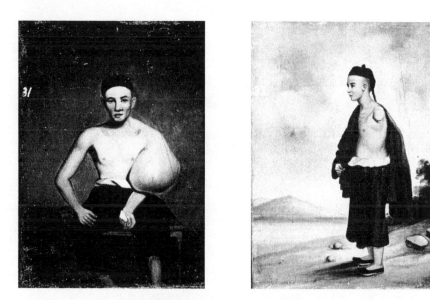

FIGURES 7 AND 8. Lam Qua, *Patient of Dr. Peter Parker (Po Ashing)*, circa 1838. Oil on canvas, 24 x 18 in. Reproduced by permission of Yale University, Harvey Cushing/ John Hay Whitney Medical Library (nos. 31 and 32 in Peter Parker Collection).

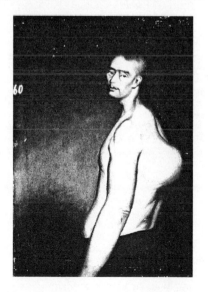

FIGURE 9. Lam Qua, *Unknown Patient of Dr. Peter Parker*, n.d. Oil on canvas, 24 x 18 in. Reproduced by permission of Yale University, Harvey Cushing/John Hay Whitney Medical Library (no. 60 in Peter Parker Collection).

Parker's surgical skill, Lam Qua's art under the pressure of medical mortality reveals itself to be what art always inevitably must be, a race against time.

NOTES

1. On the sex of this hitherto unidentified patient, see Larissa N. Heinrich, "Handmaids to the Gospel: Lam Qua's Medical Portraiture," in *Tokens of Exchange: The Problem of Translation in Global Circulations*, ed. Lydia H. Liu (Durham, NC: Duke University Press, 1999), 239–75, 272–3. Curatorial notes that inventory the collection at Yale are more equivocal, suggesting that the figure could be either male or female. Peter Josyph reproduced this image in the catalog that accompanied the only exhibition of the paintings with the gender-neutral title "Patient of Peter Parker, by Lam Qua." See Josyph, *From Yale to Canton: The Transcultural Challenge of Lam Qua and Peter Parker* [Exhibition catalog] (Smithtown, NY: Smithtown Township Arts Council, 1992), 5, 9. I will argue in this essay that the patient is a female patient named Leäng Yen.

2. While rarely seen by the public or scholars, the bulk of the paintings (eighty-six) are housed in the Peter Parker Collection in the secured storage of the Yale University Medical Historical Library and twenty-three hang in the Gordon Museum, part of Guy's Hospital in London. Four belong to Cornell University and one to the Peabody Essex Museum in Salem, Mass.

3. Thomas Colledge, Peter Parker, and Elijah C. Bridgman, "Suggestions for the Formation of a Medical Missionary Society Offered to the Consideration of all Christian Nations, More Especially to the Kindred Nations of England and the United States of America" (Canton: Medical Missionary Society in China, 1836): 8. This strategy paralleled that of seventeenth-century Jesuits who used Western astronomy for the same purpose. See Jonathan D. Spence, *To Change China: Western Advisers in China 1620–1960* (New York: Penguin Books, 1969), 34–5.

4. Osmond Tiffany, *The Canton Chinese, or the American's Sojourn in the Celestial Empire* (Boston: James Monroe, 1849), 85.

5. On perception and power, see Michel Foucault, *Discipline and Punish: The Birth of the Prison*, trans. Alan Sheridan (New York: Vintage Books, 1979), 200–1. On seeing and medicine, see Foucault, *The Birth of the Clinic: An Archaeology of Medical Perception*, trans. Alan M. Sheridan Smith (New York: Vintage Books, 1975), 107–24.

6. While not well known in general these are some of the more significant examples of nineteenth-century medical and scientific representation. On Rogue's Galleries, see Marmaduke B. Sampson, *Rationale of Crime, and Its Appropriate Treatment*, ed. Eliza Farnham (New York: D. Appleton, 1846). On Hugh Welch Diamond, see Sander L. Gilman ed., *The Face of Madness: Hugh W. Diamond and the Origin of Psychiatric Photography* (New York: Brunner/Mazel, 1976). For a discussion of Zealy's Studies, see Alan Trachtenberg, *Reading American Photographs: Images as History Mathew Brady to Walker Evans* (New York: Hill and Wang, 1989), 52–60. On medical photography, see Stanley B. Burns, *A Morning's Work: Medical Photographs from the Burns Archive and Collection, 1843–1939* (Santa Fe, NM: Twin Palms, 1998).

7. Mikhail Bakhtin, *Rabelais and His World*, trans. Helene Iswolsky (Cambridge: MIT Press, 1968), esp. 19–58 and 303–67. By "cultural grotesque" I wish to emphasize the ways in which the execution, circumstances of production, and potential meanings of Lam Qua's paintings document surprising cultural confluence.

8. Edward V. Gulick, *Peter Parker and the Opening of China* (Cambridge: Harvard University Press, 1973), 146. Gulick remarks on Parker's surgical skill despite having

large farmer's hands. On Lam Qua, see Rebecca Kinsman Munroe, "Life in Macao in the 1840s. Letters of Rebecca Chase Kinsman to her family in Salem," *Essex Institute Historical Collections* 86 (1950): 39.

9. From an 1837 letter by Parker quoted in George B. Stevens, *The Life, Letters, and Journals of the Rev. and Hon. Peter Parker, M.D., Missionary, Physician, and Diplomatist, The Father of Medical Missions and Founder of the Ophthalmic Hospital in Canton* (Boston: Congregational Sunday-School and Publishing Society, 1896), 132–3.

10. The most authoritative accounts of Lam Qua's career are Patrick Conner, "Lamqua: Western and Chinese Painter," *Arts of Asia* 29, no. 2 (1999): 46–64; and Carl L. Crossman, *The Decorative Arts of the China Trade* (Woodbridge, England: Antique Collector's Club, 1991), 72–105.

11. For overviews, see Conner, 58; and Crossman, 77–80. For specific accounts, see M. de la Vollée, "Art in China," *Bulletin of the American Art Union* (October 1850): 118–9; Paul Emile Daurand Forgues [Old Nick, pseud.], *La Chine Ouverte* (Paris: H. Fournier, 1845), 56; and William Fane de Salis, *Reminiscences of Travels in China and India in 1848* (London: Waterlow and Sons, 1892), 12. For another account, see Joachim Hounau [Georges Bell], *Voyage en Chine du Capitaine Montfort avec un résumé historique des événements des dix dernieres années* (Paris: Libraire Nouvelle, 1860), 92–107; and C. Toogood Downing, *The Fan-Qui in China, 1836–7* (London: H. Colburn, 1838), 2:91–117.

12. Munroe, 39.

13. Algernon Graves, *The Royal Academy of Arts: A Complete Dictionary of Contributors and their Work from its Foundation* (London: H. Graves, 1905–06), 4:361; Conner, 61; Crossman, 81–3; and Mary Bartlett Cowdrey, *American Academy of Fine Arts and American Art-Union: Exhibition Record 1816–1852*9 (New York: New York Historical Society, 1953), 220.

14. John Thomson, *China and Its People in Early Photographs: An Unabridged Reprint of the Classic 1873–4 Work* (New York: Dover Publications, 1982), 1: Plate IV.

15. A story was widely maintained that Lam Qua had been a houseboy and learned Western painting under Chinnery's tutelage, but Chinnery always denied this. Lam Qua may have come from a family of artists (his brother, who went by the name of Tingqua, also had a successful studio specializing in miniatures and sketches). For a summary of views see Conner, 49–54; and Crossman, 72–104.

16. Conner, 57.

17. M. de la Vollée, 119. This was expressed subtly, even in positive reports such as Rebecca Chase Kinsman's comment, "Would that I could give you an idea of the artist 'Lamqua'—A more perfect contrast to our [Salem portrait painter, Charles] Osgood can hardly be imagined. He is very *fat* and no one could imagine on looking at him, that he possessed a spark of genius, though he has in reality a great deal" (Munroe, 39). Because the corpulent Lam Qua did not conform to Kinsman's romantic ideal of the lean, intense painter, his genius was not readily perceived.

18. Ibid. See, also, Fitch W. Taylor, *A Voyage around the World* (New York: D. Appleton, 1848), 2:166. This volume reproduces many of the stock views and portraits of the emperor that Lam Qua's studio sold in great numbers.

19. "Jargon Spoken at Canton," *Chinese Repository* (January 1836): 432–3. All subsequent references to this monthly will be noted as *CR*.

20. Ibid., 433.

21. On *yi* see, Lydia H. Liu, "Legislating the Universal: The Circulation of International Law in the Nineteenth Century," in Liu, *Tokens of Exchange: The Problem of Translation in Global Circulations*, 127 64, esp. 131 5. Examples of *Fan Kwae* include William Hunter, *The "Fan-Kwae," at Canton before Treaty Days, 1825–1844* (Shanghai: Kelly and Walsh, 1911). See also the American Downing and the French Paul Emile Daurand Forgues who, by styling himself as "Old Nick," embraces this devilish moniker.

22. Colledge et al., 3–5 (italics in original).

23. Gulick, 57–8.

24. Colledge et al., 6 (italics in original).

25. Stevens, 328–9.

26. *CR* (February 1836): 466.

27. Parker only mentions the paintings once in his case notes (*CR* May 1837: 39). William Lockhart, an English medical missionary and colleague of Parker, suggests that Lam Qua painted them "to show his appreciation of the value of the Canton hospital to his countrymen." Lockhart, *The Medical Missionary in China: A Narrative of Twenty Years' Experience* (London: Hurst and Blackett, 1861), 171.

28. *CR* (May 1837): 39. "Cutting" would be in this case Pidgin English for surgery, hence Parker's use of quotations marks.

29. "Minutes of Two Annual Meetings of the Medical Missionary Society in China" (Canton, 1852): 38.

30. Article six of the regulations indicates that the "museum of natural and morbid anatomy" would include "paintings of extraordinary diseases, &c." "Medical Missionary Society: Regulations and Resolutions," *CR* (May 1838): 34.

31. Lockhart, 171. Lockhart erroneously reports that the portraits in general first show "the malady from which they suffered, and then the appearance after the patient was cured." There is only one instance in the collection of a before-and-after sequence, namely that of Po Ashing, which is in the collection at Guy's and doubtless inspired the comment. However, by giving the impression of a whole series of pre- and postoperative images, Lockhart gives the collection a more coherent medical rationale than the series actually possesses.

32. Josyph, 5, claims that Parker displayed these paintings widely during his travels in 1840–1, but I have found less evidence of this. For one account of Parker exhibiting the paintings, see *Boston Medical and Surgical Journal* 24, no. 9 (1841): 177.

33. *CR* (March 1848): 133.

34. Parker's hospital reports are dotted with these testimonials. For example, here is Parker's translation of a scroll: "Sie Kienhang of the Province of Kwangsi, presents his respects the very benevolent Dr. Parker and moved by polite attention, addresses to him the following sentiments:

'One book of healing wisdom he to regions far imparts,
And thousand verdant orange trees by the fountain's side he plants.'"
Parker, *Report of the Ophthalmic Hospital at Canton for the years 1850 and 1851* (Canton, 1852), 26–7.

35. Gulick, 125–43.

36. Stevens, 236–7.

37. Sander L. Gilman, "Lam Qua and the Development of a Westernized Medical Iconography in China," *Medical History* 30, no. 1 (1986): 57–69, 65.

38. *CR* (May 1837): 38–9.

39. For example, in some of the curatorial annotations in the collection there are notes on whether or not a particular face looks Chinese.

40. Not a prop that becomes the appurtenance of class identity, as Gilman might have it, but as a part of the body that has become a thing apart.

41. *CR* (June 1838): 99–102.

42. Ibid., 103–5.

43. The following is derived from Parker's case notes *CR* (March 1839): 576–9. Subsequent references are cited parenthetically in the text.

44. Heinrich, 273. For a similar comment on a painting of a different patient see Spence, 44.

45. Parker does not mention this in the case but in his introduction to the quarterly report. *CR* (March 1839): 569.

46. During this same period, great concern was expressed in Great Britain and America over the use of bodies for medical teaching, research, and experimentation, especially in the wake of the public outrage at the discovery of the crimes of William Burke and William Hare in 1827, who sold the corpses of the people they murdered to an anatomist. See Roy Porter, *The Greatest Benefit to Mankind: A Medical History of Mankind* (New York: W. W. Norton, 1999), esp. 317–8.

47. Michael Sullivan, *The Meeting of Eastern and Western Art* (Berkeley: University of California Press, 1989), 86.

48. The record offers some indication of Lam Qua's commitment to the mass production of stereotypical images. When it came to landscapes of Canton, Lam Qua was not particularly interested in keeping his images current. In 1850, an English observer complained that Lam Qua's studio indifferently continued to churn out views of Canton that contained the English hong, which had burned down during the opium wars. See de la Vollée, 119.

Loss and the Persistence of Memory: "The Case of George Dedlow" and Disabled Civil War Veterans

Robert I. Goler

Late in 1866, the United States Army Hospital for Injuries and Diseases of the Nervous System located on the outskirts of Philadelphia (commonly known as "Stump Hospital" by the many amputees who resided within) began receiving unsolicited financial contributions. At the same time, groups of visitors knocked on its doors requesting audiences with Dr. George Dedlow, a quadruple amputee from the Civil War whose account had recently been published in the *Atlantic Monthly*.[1]

These visitors and donors were fascinated by the first-person account of Dedlow's transformation from an assistant surgeon with the Tenth Indiana Volunteers to "a useless torso, more like some strange larval creature than anything of human shape" (5). Dedlow describes how he is wounded and captured while lost behind enemy lines. Once he is transported to an Atlanta hospital, his arm is amputated, greatly relieving his painful anguish, and he is moved to a northern hospital. Upon returning to active duty he is injured again, this time in the legs. He undergoes another surgery and upon recovering his senses in a hospital bed, he narrates, "[the attendant] threw off the covers, and, to my horror, showed me that I had suffered amputation of both thighs, very high up" (5). While in the hospital, he contracts a gangrenous infection and loses his other arm. Unable to wear prostheses, "as the stump was always too tender to bear any pressure," Dedlow exists in a liminal state contemplating his fate (5). He discusses the pain and deadened sensations associated with his "phantom limbs" and his reliance on the assistance of hospital attendants for every bodily need, including the transcription of his account. One day Dedlow overhears a fellow patient discussing his spiritualist beliefs and agrees to join him for a visit to a medium. Dedlow participates in a séance, at which he expresses his skepticism by attempting to call up his departed legs. Suddenly, the medium communicates the message she receives: "United States Army Medical Museum, Nos. 3486, 3487." "Good gracious!" shouts Dedlow, "They are *my legs*! *my legs*!" He then proceeds to rise, staggering across the room "on limbs invisible to them or me." After this brief caper, Dedlow "fainted and rolled over senseless." The account ends with him retired, drawing a government pension and awaiting death (11).

"The Case of George Dedlow," a fictional and, at times, tongue-in-cheek account (the legs stagger because they have been kept for several months in a vat of alcohol) was published in the guise of an autobiographical essay. Its true author, S. Weir Mitchell (1829–1914), later became known as an eminent medical specialist, originator of the "rest cure" for women, and author. Though a fictional character, Dedlow was intensely real to his would-be visitors, who flatly refused to believe the superintendent of "Stump Hospital" when he explained that Dedlow did not live there.[2]

Dedlow's admirers, while misguided, can hardly be blamed for believing the lurid account of suffering and the supernatural. Much about the postwar experience must have seemed unreal to many Americans. By the time Generals Robert E. Lee and Ulysses S. Grant met at Appomattox, Virginia, to sign terms of surrender in April 1865, over six hundred thousand men had died and another five hundred thousand were injured. Americans had never witnessed suffering on such a brutal, violent, and massive scale.[3] After this traumatic experience, hundreds of thousands of veterans on both sides of the Mason-Dixon Line returned to their homes hoping to reconstruct their lives, but many were never the same. These men had experienced deprivation, had watched comrades fall in battle and languish from disease, and had seen the landscape and built environment ravished. Having seen the unforgettable, they were scarred, emotionally and physically, for life. Noncombatants also found themselves struggling to accept the physical and emotional changes in their fathers, husbands, and brothers. Across America, those who returned with amputated limbs were an extraordinarily visible group. These veterans provoked a profound mixture of love and horror, fascination and anxiety.

This essay explores the representations of the experience and medical treatment of those whose limbs were amputated as a result of battlefield injuries. In addition to examining their medical records, I investigate examples of the photography that documented the unparalleled suffering of severely injured veterans. My essay has three complementary trajectories: first, analyzing the trauma generated by the Civil War; second, addressing questions of identity that emerged for Civil War amputees; and, finally, discerning some of the cultural meanings attributed to the Civil War's many disabled veterans. D. J. Canale's review of S. Weir Mitchell's medical career in the Civil War suggests that "The Case of George Dedlow" may have been intended as a testimonial to the terrible losses suffered by field surgeons at the Battle of Gettysburg.[4] While usually viewed by medical historians and physicians as a speculative essay on neurology and "phantom limb" syndrome, "The Case of George Dedlow" also contains important information about the emergence of attitudes toward a new social category: the disabled.[5] In its interrelation of national trauma, personal trauma, and the symbolic role assigned veteran amputees in the search for communal suture, "The Case of George Dedlow" exemplifies these three trajectories. Ultimately, however, the veteran amputee resists such attempts at repair. Embodying loss, the Civil War veteran amputee remained an ambiguous figure, simultaneously epitomizing survival and death, victory and bereavement.

Disability and the Civil War

Historians often characterize the Civil War as the first modern war because of the ferocity of its devastation and the degree to which it was given realistic and nearly contemporary representation in print and visual media. Photography, which emerged as a form of documentary journalism for the first time in the mid-nineteenth century, created greater public awareness of the realities of battlefields littered with corpses. These images, quickly reproduced and distributed to those wishing to compile "albums of war," appeared nationally, accompanying newspaper accounts.[6]

On the battlefields, surgeons from both Union and Confederate armies struggled to keep pace with the injuries. With over seven million cases of disease treated and more than two hundred and fifty thousand wounds examined on the Union side alone, the impetus to develop new strategies for medical treatment was intense. Of particular concern were the large gashes and shattered bones caused by the minié ball, a newly introduced conical bullet whose force and velocity dramatically changed the nature of gunshot wounds. Most notable among these injuries were the thirty thousand amputations that required quick resolution of a ruined limb if the soldier was to survive under the rough conditions of

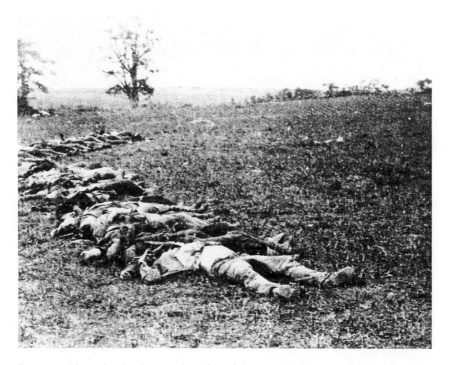

FIGURE 1. Alexander Gardner, *Bodies of Confederate Dead at Antietam*, 1862. Library of Congress.

battlefield surgery. The majority of these procedures were of fingers or the hand; however, large numbers of shoulder, elbow, knee, and hip amputations also had to be performed. Most operations were over within two minutes, including the time needed to close off arteries and prepare a covering skin flap. Limited awareness of modern sanitary methods partly caused the high mortality rates, particularly for amputations.[7]

Recognizing the terrible toll of these injuries, Dr. William Hammond, the Union army's surgeon general, called for a systematic documentation of battlefield wounds for study at the Medical Department. This type of scientific approach to documenting battlefield medical conditions had been attempted by both the French and the British at Sebastopol, during the Crimean War, but both efforts had failed to follow postoperative conditions.[8] To remedy this deficiency, United States Army doctors were enlisted to gather specimens to be sent to a central repository for preservation and future study. Record keeping became integral to the Medical Department's efforts; several overlapping means of compiling information were developed to transcribe and organize surgical notes. In the case of amputation or excision, the severed limb itself was forwarded to Washington for study. Specimens previously saved at military hospitals across the country were also shipped to Washington, including limbs that had been severed, samples of injured internal organs, and surgically removed tissues. John Brinton, curator of the new Army Medical Museum, established in Washington in 1862, issued protocols for collecting specimens and traveled the eastern battlefields to meet surgeons and observe fresh injuries. Specimens were to be cleaned, tagged, and then "packed away in a keg, containing alcohol, whiskey, or sometimes salt and water" until the keg was full and could be shipped to Washington where the specimens would undergo final preparation before being placed on the shelves. The memoranda or histories of these specimens were in the meantime forwarded to the surgeon general's office and, after being verified and affixed to their rightful objects, were entered in the books of *Histories of Specimens*.[9] Within the first few months, seven thousand specimens were assembled. Over time, the collection of amputated limbs and shrapnel expanded to include medical equipment, photographs, and weapons.[10] As a result, for the first time in recorded history, a large body of scientific specimens from military battlefields was assembled, complete with accompanying documentation.

In addition to collecting documentary and physical evidence of battlefield amputations, the Medical Department initiated procedures to develop photographic records of specimens and patients, including long-term follow-up documentation of postoperative veterans. Already, before the war, photographic medical records had been introduced, as selected images of medical anomalies had been distributed among physicians and medical societies. As a contributor to the *Photographic Journal* commented, "[T]he day is not far hence when the museum of every medical school will be furnished with photographic illustrations of the terribly diversified forms of disease [that] . . . do not depend on the lively imagination of the lithographer."[11] With the onset of the Civil War this prediction quickly became reality. It was the first large-scale conflict in which medically significant numbers of injuries were recorded photographically.

The Army Medical Museum welcomed this new use of photography. Established by the army's surgeon general, the museum was intended to be a repository of battlefield injuries encompassing "all specimens of morbid anatomy, surgical or medical . . . together with projectiles and foreign bodies removed."[12] This institution was the first

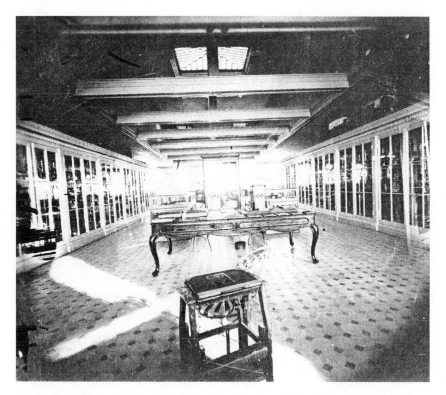

FIGURE 2. Attributed to William Bell, *Main Gallery, Army Medical Museum*, 1867. National Museum of Health and Medicine.

to effectively combine medical photography with military conflict. Its location in the same building as the Pension and Records Division and the Surgeon General's Library reinforced Hammond's attempts to catalogue battlefield injuries.

The photographs of injured veterans served both medical and political purposes. First, after being catalogued and examined at the Army Medical Museum, the images were copied and published in a series of volumes entitled *Surgical Photographs* and then distributed to medical schools and military installations to assist in training for military medicine. Second, veterans who provided full documentation of their injuries (often including obligatory photographs) were eligible to be fitted for prostheses and to receive monthly payments.[13] In his discussion of other patients in one of the many hospitals he visited, the fictional Dedlow recalls a "tall, blond-bearded major [who] . . . exposed

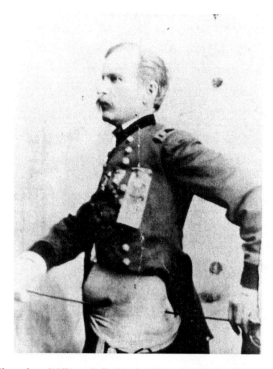

FIGURE 3. Attributed to William Bell, *Musket Wound of Major Henry A. Barnum*, 1865. National Museum of Health and Medicine.

his left hip[:] `Ball went in here, and out here'" (4). It is possible that Mitchell had in mind Major Henry A. Barnum (Twelfth New York), who was wounded by a musket ball at Malvern Hill in 1862.[14] Because Barnum's wound never healed, he was able to pull a skein through the wound to permit regular drainage. Despite this remarkable condition, Barnum returned to battle and rose to the rank of major general. In subsequent years, Barnum returned to Washington to have new photographs taken of his wound as visual support for petitions to Congress to increase his pension.

Photographs, such as those of Barnum, compiled for purposes of medical investigation and pension records, form a body of haunting, evocative images. Depicting the human cost of war with a harsh directness, the photographs plainly show the loss that "was more difficult to see and acknowledge than the grisly remains of corpses soon transfigured into stone monuments": the ravaged bodies of those still among the living.[15] "The Case of George Dedlow," playing on the exhibitionism of veterans like Barnum, must have struck a chord for many citizens who were only now for the first time encountering severely injured veterans.

From Trauma to Narrative

"The distance between self and other is always disturbed," writes Geoffrey Hartman. "There is always some difficulty of self-presentation in us . . . [and] we are obliged to fall back on a form of 'representa-tion.'"[16] Representations of the traumatic wounding of veterans in both archival sources (the army repositories) and literature (as illustrated by "The Case of George Dedlow") became a form of coping and enabled identity re-formation in post–Civil War America. In particular, the development of the photographic archive, as well as the display of severed limbs in the Army Medical Museum, sharply focus our atten-tion on the interface between subject and viewer and compel us to pose these questions: How are soldiers changed by war, and how are these changes perceived and interpreted by others? To what extent does the wounded veteran retain individual personhood in the eyes of the viewer—and of the nation—and to what extent is the veteran reflexively transformed into a symbol, whether of courage or of tragedy? How does personal trauma recapitulate social trauma, and how do healing and the limits of healing affect the body politic?

Underlying all the written and visual discourse surrounding the veteran amputees, the primary fact of injury remains: the veteran amputee bears a permanent and often permanently visible wound. "The main purpose and outcome of war," writes Elaine Scarry in *The Body in Pain*, "is injuring."[17] Scarry argues that wound making is not incidental, but central to war and that injuring the enemy serves two distinct functions. First, it "serves as a basis for a contest" by demon-strating one side's victory over the other. Second, the declaration of victory "provides a source of substantiation" for the cause undertaken by the winning side. The infliction of wounds tangibly manifests victory: the loser bears a literal stigma—the *stigmata* of defeat. The infliction of injury, the branding of the enemy's flesh, extends hege-mony by displaying the victor's dominance. Because the infliction of injury functions as a primary signifier of victory, the post–Civil War presence of thousands of permanently injured, victorious Union veter-ans created a disturbing disjunction: the very men whose lives (or worthy deaths) were expected to exemplify victory and dominance carried on their bodies indelible inscriptions of loss.

This disjunction underscores the ways in which wartime radically alters the relationship between the individual and the state. While the state can compel individuals to enlist in military service, this process implies reciprocal responsibilities between the state and its citizens. From the beginning of the American republic, the United States has compensated disabled military veterans and their families. In addition to making financial payments, the government in the early nineteenth century began a program of providing long-term housing for disabled and aging veterans.

Following the Civil War, the sheer volume of claims from Union veterans (disabled Confederates were not entitled to compensation) absorbed substantial national resources. In the year ending June 1866, for example, the Pension and Records Division examined and classified 210,027 disability discharges and provided information on another 49,212 cases to the Pension Bureau and other offices. Between 1865 and 1870 the government spent more funds on veterans than it had, cumulatively, in the preceding eighty years.[18] Veterans applying for disability benefits were required to submit evidence of their injury, documenting the circumstances under which the injury occurred and submitting affidavits from witnesses and a current medical examination report. Examiners at the Pension and Records Division then reviewed this evidence. In time their recommendations were reviewed by congressional officials, who rendered a decision. In the final decades of the century, as veterans' lobbying groups and politicians eager to dispense patronage gained influence, the requirements for proving injury were revised until, ultimately, evidence of military service itself was alone considered sufficient for compensation.[19] In addition to the paperwork requirements, veterans were occasionally asked to submit photographs of their injuries along with affidavits from examining physicians. Some veterans, such as Major General Barnum, used every available opportunity to have photographs of their wounds forwarded to Congress in the hopes of having their pensions increased. Such photographs and records were added to the research files at the Army Medical Museum. Over time, this process of collecting and expanding Civil War veteran case histories generated a substantial body of evidence documenting the diversity and long-term effects of wartime injury. In 1887, the Army Medical Museum moved to the National Mall, where many of the photographs and preserved limbs remained on view. In 1968, the collection was removed from public view, and when it was redisplayed on the grounds of the Walter Reed Army Medical Center in the mid-1970s, the more graphic examples of surgical photographs and pathology specimens had been gradually removed to storage.[20]

Scarry's idea that the aim of war is actual wounding helps us to explore how these medical representations of Civil War veterans articulate the relationship between the victorious state and its injured citizens. According to Scarry, wounding the enemy is the essential project of war, to which all other aims (such as emancipating slaves) are subordinated. The Army Medical Museum's massive archives and photographs of permanently wounded veterans, then, represent a peculiar kind of stock taking on the part of the state, for instead of participating in the celebration and institutionalization of victory, they represent a documenting of its wounds. The amputee photographs at the Army Medical Museum are, as Alan Trachtenberg remarks, "the most unforgettable of the albums of war. They disclose the most immediate and least comprehensible of war's facts, that it is waged on tangible human flesh and inscribed in pain—the living wounded body as the final untellable legend."[21] The simultaneous intensity and detached objectivity make the images startling and disturbing. The photographs underscore the individual suffering experienced by these men without giving the solace associated with war memorials. Perhaps this explains why they have remained relatively unknown.

Their ambiguous relationship to late-nineteenth-century aesthetic conventions makes these images even more disturbing. James T. H. Connor and Michael Rhode have noted that the style of the veteran photographs differs little from the style of photographs produced by professional photography studios of the era.[22] The men, sometimes naked or partially draped in sheets, and sometimes exposing only the stumps of their limbs, sit or stand in the poses of conventional portraiture, leaning on upholstered chairs and set against an ornamental backdrop of drapery. An almost grotesque tension results between the horrific wounds and the placid domestic settings in which they are displayed. The incongruity of placing exposed stumps and naked men into an imagined drawing room underscores the uncertain state of the disabled within America in the years following the Civil War. The permanently injured veteran was at once the object of anxiety, the object of attempts to "normalize" his condition, and the object of bureaucratic cataloguing. "Civil War photography," argues Timothy Sweet, "proscribed any representation of the borderline between life and death." Sweet's generalization, however, applies to the realm of photography intended for public consumption. The vast archive of medical portraiture documents the reality apparent to disabled veterans and the communities among whom they lived, but the archive was available primarily to medical researchers and received scant attention from the photographers and writers engaged in interpreting the war for the public. "The dead," says Sweet, "were fit subjects of memorialization . . . but the wounded were not to be memorialized."[23] While not memorialized, these veterans were meticulously, perhaps even obsessively, archived.

The photographic images of amputees constitute a silent dialogue on the trauma experienced by the injured veteran and the state. Unlike the cleaned, numbered, and often anonymous limbs in the cases of the Army Medical Museum, these photographs depict recognizable individuals. And they suggest a remarkably reciprocal relationship between subject and object: the direct gaze of the subject meets the gaze of the observer. The "detachment" of those unabashed poses and the detachment of those cataloguing disabilities speak to the photographs' status as "clinical legend[s]."[24]

George Dedlow: Phantom Limb and the Persistence of Memory

The experience represented by the medical histories, photographs, and severed limbs of the Army Medical Museum—the objectified experience of the disabled Civil War veteran—is given powerful literary expression in "The Case of George Dedlow." Like the subjects of the surgical photographs, Dedlow is part hero, part grotesque curiosity. As with the subjects of the photographs, Dedlow is both intensely individual and at the same time deprived of his subjectivity. In fact, Dedlow actually loses his own sense of subjectivity as a result of the medical procedures that have both saved and diminished him. "I found to my horror that at times I was less conscious of myself, of my own existence, than used to be the case. This sensation was so novel, that at first it quite bewildered me. I felt like asking some one constantly if I were really George Dedlow or not; . . . It was . . . a deficiency in the egotistic sentiment of individuality" (8). The process of dismemberment correspondingly erases his sense of personhood. Dedlow documents the disappearance of his subjectivity through a curiously detached medical analysis of the phenomenon: "About one half of the sensitive surface of my skin was gone, and thus much of relation to the outer world destroyed. As a consequence, a large part of the receptive central organs must be out of employ, and, like other idle things, degenerating rapidly. Moreover, all the great central ganglia . . . were also eternally at rest" (8). Ironically, the very diminution of his physical and psychological presence gives rise to his literary presence: he writes to the general public in order to describe and document his own eclipse. And, in addition to documenting his medical "research" on himself, he wishes to consider its psychological implications: "This set me to thinking how much a man might lose and yet live" (8). Dedlow's account is a study of loss and the transformation of identity.

S. Weir Mitchell, the author of "The Case of George Dedlow," had recently served as a surgeon at Philadelphia's Turner Hospital, an army hospital specializing in neurological disorders. A native of Philadelphia, Mitchell received a medical degree from Jefferson Medical College before spending two years in Paris studying with the renowned experimental biologist Claude Bernard. Following a decade in private practice, Mitchell enlisted in the Union forces at the outbreak of the Civil War and was assigned to surgical duties at a local military hospital. There he "began to be interested in cases of nervous disease and wounds of nerves, about which little was . . . known."[25]

This interest prompted him to propose that the army establish in Philadelphia a special hospital for nervous disorders. When the facility opened in 1862, Mitchell undertook extensive research leading to his first important medical publication, *Gunshot Wounds and Other Injuries of Nerves* (1864), which detailed findings made on soldiers under the hospital's care.[26] From his work with amputees in the army hospital, Mitchell found evidence that many continued to have sensations associated with limbs that had been removed. Mitchell's interests in this topic led to his next major publication, *Injuries of the Nerves and Their Consequences* (1872), in which he explores the characteristics that distinguish individuals who suffer phantom limb pain from those who do not. His findings correlated the phenomenon with the amount of preamputation pain the soldier had experienced.

"The Case of George Dedlow," written in the midst of this research and drafted as a private meditation on the dilemmas of identity, corporeality, and trauma, interrogates the same phenomena Mitchell was examining scientifically at the hospital ward.[27] The fictional Dr. Dedlow, who elaborates on the various nervous conditions associated with amputation as part of what "I have seen in my practice of medicine," is, literally, Mitchell's ghostwriter (6). In his scientific writing Mitchell had consistently adopted the deterministic principles he learned from Bernard, who believed all physiological phenomena had materialist origins. Yet the wealth of phantom limb observations Mitchell encountered in the army hospitals sparked a covert interest in seemingly inexplicable medical phenomena. Perhaps the conflict between Bernard's principles and his interest in phantom limbs prompted Mitchell to present his thoughts in the disguise of fiction in "The Case of George Dedlow."[28]

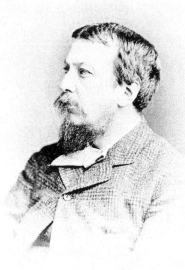

FIGURE 4. F. Gutekunst, *S. Weir Mitchell, M.D.*, 1878. Reproduced by permission of the New York Academy of Medicine Library.

"The Case of George Dedlow" represented Mitchell's attempt to excavate the psychological implications of his scientific research. He wrote the account in response to an inquiry from a friend: "How much of a man would have to be lost in order that he should lose any portion of his sense of individuality?"[29] Mitchell claimed that the story was sent without his knowledge to the publisher of the *Atlantic Monthly*.[30] Like the Army Medical Museum's *Surgical Photographs*, which began as an internal project for medical instruction and later were displayed in public galleries where they shocked and fascinated visitors, "Dedlow" originated in Mitchell's private circle but caused a public sensation.

In "The Case of George Dedlow," Mitchell uses the compositional freedoms of fiction and pseudonymity to explore what could not be discussed in medical journals. The text addresses ambiguous and conflicting evidence on amputation, particularly phantom limbs, in a manner that allows him to express his scientific findings without the strictures of scientific discourse. Dedlow prefaces his story with a disclaimer; these accounts, he says, have been declined "by every medical journal to which I have offered them." Indeed, he says, the story is "not of any scientific value whatsoever" but of metaphysical value (1).

Mitchell begins Dedlow's account by establishing the narration as both sympathetic and trustworthy. The son of a midwestern village doctor, Dedlow's medical studies were interrupted by the outbreak of the war. Volunteering for service, he was appointed an assistant surgeon in a regiment that was quickly decimated. Reassigned to a new regiment and posted near Nashville, his life, like other Civil War soldiers, was "tedious, and at the same time dangerous in the extreme. Food was scarce and bad, the water horrible," and the locals hostile (2).

Sent out alone on a special mission, Dedlow is injured, captured, and sent to a confederate hospital near Atlanta. Dedlow gives a graphic description of the agony caused by his inflamed right arm. Commenting to a hospital visitor that his hand is now "dead except to pain," he is the recipient of an impromptu sermon to the effect that "such and thus will the wicked be—such will you be if you die in your sins: . . . [A]ll of you will be as that hand,—knowing pain only" (3). This remarkable theological peroration is immediately followed by an account of the surgical removal of Dedlow's arm without benefit of anesthesia. He reports that the pain of the operation, while great, was "insignificant" compared with the pain of the infected limb or with the relief brought by amputation. Then, he says, "I slept,—slept the sleep of the just, or, better, of the painless" (4). The account of Dedlow's first amputation provides a vivid foreshadowing of the themes Mitchell raises later in the story. The stranger identifies the pain of the injured limb with damnation, an experience of "knowing pain only." Dedlow's own account that, separated from his pain (that is, his arm), he slept the sleep of "the just or, better, of the painless," reinforces the impression that pain represents damnation while relief, brought about by the limb's absence, is literally a blessed condition. Dedlow must lose the arm and its pain in order to achieve moral wholeness. Seeing the severed arm on the hospital floor, he comments, "There is the pain, and here am I" (4). Dedlow's narrative effectively defines amputation as a *positive* experience, a condition that carries not only medical but also spiritual benefits. Moreover, Dedlow claims that his own experience is representative: "[A]t a subsequent period I saw a number of cases similar to mine in a hospital in Philadelphia" (4). Dedlow's readers also knew of cases similar to his, in the persons of friends and family members maimed from the war. But whereas the civilian population had little means to comprehend the experience of these individuals, Dedlow positioned himself as a spokesperson for that deeply ambiguous citizen in America, the disabled veteran.

At this stage in his narrative, Dedlow has established the disabled veteran, as exemplified by himself, as a heroic, even a redeemed figure. After suffering both hardship and injury for his country, he has literally sacrificed a part of himself and by virtue of that sacrifice has been saved from the living hell of ceaseless pain. Mitchell, through Dedlow, seems fully to embrace the suturing process through which survival is transmuted into heroism and injury into a "badge of courage." The narrative now takes a curious turn. Following a second traumatic injury, Dedlow loses both his legs and his remaining arm. Rather than sleeping the sleep of the just/painless, he becomes an object of "anguish and horror" to himself. Instead of detailing his own anguish, however, Dedlow addresses himself to his purported goal: "to possess [his reader] with facts in regard to the relation of the mind to the body" (5). Dedlow proceeds to describe in great detail the experience now known as "phantom limb," a subject of Mitchell's ongoing research among army veterans. After discussing the sensation "felt" by his own missing limbs, Dr. Dedlow gives a scientific account of the phenomenon. The perception of sensation, he says, arises only while the severed nerves are in the process of healing. When the healing is completed, the sensations cease: "[I]n a very healthy stump, no such impressions arise." In some cases, however, including Dedlow's own, "a more or less constant irritation of the nerve-fibres" develops, with the result that the brain "preserves to the man a consciousness of possessing that which he has not" (6). The *illusion* of wholeness represented by phantom limb sensations is in fact symptomatic of a *lack* of wholeness, that is, of an injury that has not healed. The persistence of memory turns out to be nothing more than the persistence of the pain associated with loss. Moreover, the promise of medical science, the redemption from pain effected by amputation, has proven illusory, since now the *illusion* of pain in the limb has taken the place of its reality.

Ironically, just as Dedlow undergoes the return of the pain he once believed he had escaped ("There is my pain, and here am I."), he begins to lose the sense of his own identity. His physical dismemberment can go no further—he has lost four-fifths of his weight, his heart has slowed to forty-five beats per minute, and he has lost a third of his skin. Now, however, the loss of external "self" precipitates a loss of subjectivity. "I thus reached the conclusion," notes Dedlow, "that a man is not his brain, or any one part of it, but all of his economy, and that to lose any part must lessen this sense of his own existence" (8). Even as Dedlow realizes the failure of medical science—both body and selfhood have become truncated by operations that have left him in the hell of "knowing nothing save pain"—he is approached by the spiritualist.

Dedlow's recourse to the séance is, of course, the antithesis of the training Mitchell had received under Bernard. But to Mitchell's readers, the séance was a tantalizingly "scientific" means of making a connection to the spiritual world. The nineteenth century had developed a passion for electricity as an entirely new means of communication. The telegraph communicated invisibly across previously unbridgeable spaces, prompting the popular appellation of "the spiritual telegraph" for séances.[31] Benjamin Franklin's remark that electricity was comprised of "disembodied spirits" and Mary Shelley's enlivening of Frankenstein's creature by means of an electrical storm expressed the popular interest in finding a connection between electrical and spiritual powers. Medical treatments using electricity, which had been in use in America since colonial times, gained in popularity in the mid-nineteenth century with the widespread availability of electrotherapy machines to stimulate muscles.[32] And the public may well have known, as Mitchell certainly did, that anatomists had experimented in the effects of applying electricity to corpses to study muscle function.[33] The very fact that Mitchell's fantastic account was widely accepted as factual testifies to a popular desire of many nineteenth-century readers to accept descriptions of electricity moving limbs. Mitchell himself, of course, held no such beliefs. In response to various spiritualist leaders who found in "Dedlow" confirmation of their methods, he responded sardonically: "Imagine that!"[34]

The account of the séance, however parodic, provides a counterweight to the lengthy descriptions of the medical procedures performed on Dedlow and the losses, both physical and psychological, that medical science proved unable to prevent. The séance within the narrative, after all, is successful. Whereas Dedlow's physical stumps caused only pain in the phantom members, the missing members themselves, now existing in a spiritual realm, arrive to carry him painlessly across the room. Even in their scientifically depersonalized state (no longer the legs of Dedlow, they are "United States Army Medical Museum, Nos. 3486, 3487"), his "spiritual" legs are better able to restore his full personhood than the surgeon's knife. "Suddenly," he recalls, "I felt a strange return of my self-consciousness. I was re-individualized, so to speak" (11). The spiritualist has performed a suture unavailable to the physician. Ultimately, however, the promise of spiritual solace, like the promise of medical solace, proves short lived: "Presently, however, I felt myself sinking slowly. My legs were going, and in a moment I was

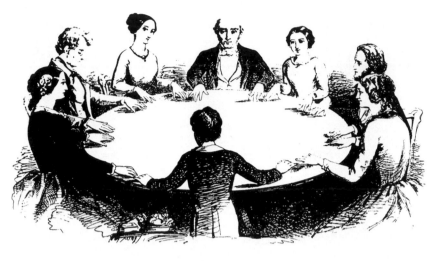

TABLE   MOVING.

FIGURE 5. Artist Unknown, *Table Moving*, circa 1860. Lithograph. Private Collection.

resting feebly on my two stumps upon the floor. It was too much. All that was left of me fainted and rolled over senseless" (11). Dedlow concludes his narrative observing that, though "surrounded by every form of kindness," he continues to suffer the loss of his sense of self and is "not a happy fraction of a man." Rather, he longs for the day "when I shall rejoin the lost members of my corporeal family in another and a happier world" (11).

"The Case of George Dedlow," a story that captivated the hearts and imaginations of many readers, melancholically and bitterly reflects on irredeemable loss. The promise of medical science has born bitter fruit. The removal of Dedlow's limbs, causing the atrophy of his very self, fails to produce the promised freedom from pain. As predicted by the hospital preacher, the only knowledge left to his legs—redefined solely as objects of scientific research—is the knowledge of pain. The spiritual route has, like the medical, offered only the briefest illusion of reintegration. In the end, he must face his life as a "fragment of a man," still awaiting a meaningful restoration. Dedlow's hope for reunion with his dearly departed limbs mirrors the experience of countless veterans who, along with the families of the deceased, formed a continual stream of visitors to Washington's Army Medical Museum. They came to glimpse, to hold, to be however fleetingly reunited with the lost limbs that represented the loss of loved ones, or, for some, of themselves.

"The Case of George Dedlow" presents a powerful example of how literature can sometimes effect cultural work outside its normal orbit. Turning to fiction enabled Mitchell to interpret his research with more creativity than would have been possible had he written solely for his medical colleagues. Lisa Herschbach, looking more broadly at Mitchell's literary output from this period, makes a similar argument, suggesting that we read "The Case of George Dedlow" as "a contrapuntal position *vis-à-vis* Mitchell's medico-scientific text[s]."[35] In "The Case of George Dedlow," Mitchell metaphorically and structurally merged his personal and professional identities, choosing to represent the phenomenological dilemma of phantom limbs in a framework that combines a case history with autobiography.

The convergence of literature and medicine did gain modest acceptance in Mitchell's lifetime. Stanley Blair has demonstrated how literary works began to appear regularly in medical journals at the turn of the twentieth century.[36] The impact of the Civil War on Mitchell's literary career cannot be overstated. "The Case of George Dedlow" was his first published work, and the Civil War was the setting for his first and last novels, *In War Time* (1884) and *Westways* (1913), respectively. Much of Mitchell's fiction was written in an autobiographical voice and set in Philadelphia. Mitchell, though, perceived literary and medical description to be different genres, and he used them for different ends. Herschbach has suggested that the strength of Mitchell's writing came from his ability to compose "contradictory and internally antagonistic" accounts in his fiction and medical works.[37] Mitchell's ability to draw upon his personal experience for "The Case of George Dedlow" allows the reader to see the social wounding caused by war. Public awareness of the medical toll of the Civil War gained greater appreciation in subsequent years but was always linked with other projects of national ascension.

Ten Years Later: Medicine on Display

At the Centennial Exposition of American Independence in Philadelphia in 1876, the United States Army constructed a model hospital to symbolize the substantial accomplishments of the medical corps in translating improvements in medical treatment to the battlefield and to offer the public a chance to see the latest advances in medical science. Among the exhibits were copies of the first few volumes of the *Medical and Surgical History of the War of the Rebellion*, the massive research project (ultimately comprising some six thousand pages) transcribing, reproducing, and analyzing data related to war injuries that had been compiled by the Medical Department.[38] To complement the *Medical and Surgical History,* a selection of the surgical photographs from the Army Medical Museum was displayed in a nearby gallery. This public display marked a radical departure from the use of these images for medical and pension record purposes alone.

The photographs, with their graphic impressions of gaunt, scarred, and mutilated soldiers, brought back to public view the stark reality of the war, but now in the festive context of an exhibit celebrating military medical advances. Officials of the Army Medical Museum, hoping to protect the sensibility of viewers rather than the privacy of the veterans, had arranged to have fig leaves painted over the exposed genitals of veterans who had posed naked.[39] The symbolic transformation of these images from representations of suffering and loss to representations of medical progress, from wounded individuals to decorously draped subjects of military pride, suggests how quickly perceptions of these woundings transformed—or at least how quickly the army sought to transform their meaning.

In the same pavilion, visitors could view the amputee photographs and illustrated medical histories as well as a massive portrait of Dr. Samuel Gross, recently completed by Thomas Eakins (figure 7). The eight-foot-tall painting portrays one of the country's leading surgeons in the midst of an operating theater, lecturing to medical students about an incision into the thigh of an anesthetized patient. Gross, a scalpel in his bloody hand, looks away from the patient and into the distance, striking a pose of dramatic heroism. The patient is visible only as an exposed buttock and thigh, the object of industrious suturing on the part of Gross's assistants. Eakins had expected the painting to hang in the art gallery, but the selection committee rejected it as being too realistic and it was instead displayed in the army's medical pavilion.[40] Eakins's painting reflects a sensibility similar to that represented in the nearby gallery of Civil War injuries. "No one who has ever stood before *The Gross Clinic,*" writes art historian Michael Fried, "needs to be reminded just how complex and disturbing are the responses that [the bloodied hand and scalpel] inevitably elicit . . . until at last it becomes apparent that something in all this must be distinctly pleasurable, which is to say that the act of looking emerges here as a source of mingled pain and pleasure, violence and voluptuousness, repulsion and fascination."[41] In both the photographs and the painting, the patients' identities have been altered or (in the case of the Eakins painting) erased altogether. In both, the glory of medical accomplishment is established

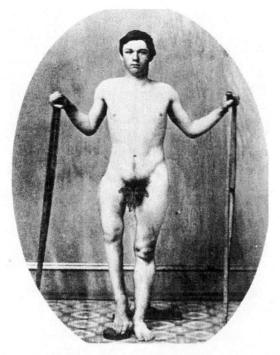

FIGURE 6. Photographer Unknown, *Excision of Right Femur on Private Jason W. Joslyn* n.d. National Museum of Health and Medicine.

by reference to the patient's visible but passive suffering (the missing limbs of the veterans and the exposed buttock of the anesthetized patient). Competition between the didactic goals of the presentation and the innate fascination of the wounded bodies appears in both exhibits. Gross, sharing the center of the canvas with the wound, is portrayed as a valorous surgeon demonstrating his prowess before the waiting crowd. As for the veterans, the culmination of their military service as specimens in the *Medical and Surgical History*—where their individual experiences and catalogued limbs were carefully compared and studied—had transformed them into symbols of traumatic experience that were superceded by the patriotic enthusiasms of the Exposition. In both cases, individual wounding is positioned to affirm the triumph of the nation.

This repositioning of the medical consequences of the Civil War did not, however, cause veterans such as Mitchell to forget the violence they had experienced. In Mitchell's rise in the ranks of Philadelphia

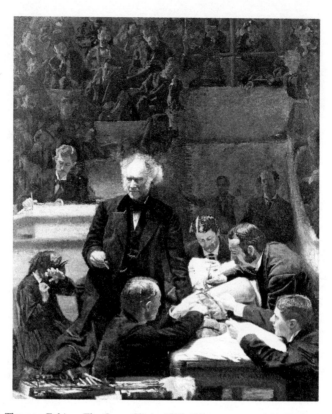

FIGURE 7. Thomas Eakins, *The Gross Clinic*, 1875. Oil on canvas, 96 x 78 in. Reproduced by permission of Jefferson Medical College of Thomas Jefferson University, Philadelphia.

society, the imprint of his years of military service during the Civil War remained. As Eakins was painting *The Gross Clinic*, Mitchell assumed two new positions of social and professional prestige. He was elected trustee of the University of Pennsylvania and appointed president of the American Neurological Association. In these capacities, and as a long-time patron of Philadelphian organizations (not to mention his status as a Civil War veteran), Mitchell surely attended the Centennial Exposition and ventured into the army pavilion. But it was not the affirmative message of the Exposition that Mitchell recalled when he reviewed his life for the final time. On his deathbed half a century after the Civil War, Mitchell returned to the painful and vivid memories of his military service: "[H]is wandering talk was of mutilation and bullets; he conversed and argued with that past."[42] For Mitchell, as for Dedlow, the traumas of bodily wounding during the Civil War continued to torture his soul.

The dismemberment and temporary reattachment that Mitchell had described in "The Case of George Dedlow" offers a potent metaphor for the suturing that Mitchell felt was necessary for the United States to rediscover its identity after the Civil War. Where Scarry claims that the process of wounding enables the state to become the soldier, Mitchell argues that soldiers, by giving their bodies to it, become the state. In this he echoed the contemporary (but unpublished) reflections of poet Walt Whitman, then a Civil War hospital aide: "The soldier drops, sinks like a wave—but the ranks of the ocean eternally press on. Death does its work, obliterates a hundred, a thousand—President, general, captain, private—but the Nation is immortal."[43] The life force represented by Dedlow's phantom limbs symbolized the integral role of disabled veterans to the health of the state. Yet, as with the fictional Dedlow, disabled veterans required care and acceptance. As the disabled political apparatus of the Southern states was to be rebuilt, so too did the injured veterans require active reconstruction. Perhaps the widespread call for charity and the omnipresence of injury and loss that pervaded the nation in the aftermath of the Civil War resonated with these subliminal aspects of Dedlow's account, prompting the readers to come to his aid.[44] For Mitchell, true patriotism resided in the care of these veterans, in repairing injury and restoring lost limbs.

NOTES

The author would like to thank the following individuals for their suggestions in the preparation of this article: Randall Bass, Julie Galambush, David Gerber, Michael O'Malley, and Michael Rhode.
1. [S. Weir Mitchell], "The Case of George Dedlow," *Atlantic Monthly* 18, no. 105 (July 1866): 1–11. A facsimile of the original imprint is available online at http://cdl.library.cornell.edu/moa/ (accessed March 30, 2004). Subsequent references are cited parenthetically in the text.
2. S. Weir Mitchell, "The Medical Department in the Civil War," *JAMA* 52, no. 19 (1914): 1445–50, 1448 [published posthumously]. The catalogue numbers given for Dedlow's legs do not match any actual collection items from the Army Medical Museum.
3. John Duffy, *The Healers: A History of American Medicine* (Urbana: University of Illinois Press, 1976), 207–10; and Anne C. Rose, *Victorian America and the Civil War* (New York: Cambridge University Press, 1992).
4. D. J. Canale, "Civil War Medicine from the Perspective of S. Weir Mitchell's 'The Case of George Dedlow,'" *Journal of the History of the Neurosciences* 11, no. 1 (2002): 17.
5. See, for example, John C. Goldner, "S. Weir Mitchell: Nerves, Peripheral and Otherwise," *Mayo Clinic Proceedings* 46 (1971): 274–81; Morton Nathanson, "Phantom

Limbs as Reported by S. Weir Mitchell," *Neurology* 38, no. 3 (1988): 504–5; and Jerome Schneck, "S. Weir Mitchell, M.D. (1829–1914): Neurologic and Psychiatric Observations in 'The Case of George Dedlow,'" *New York State Journal of Medicine* 79, no. 11 (1979): 1777–82.

6. On the history of Civil War photography and its uses see Timothy Sweet, *Traces of War: Poetry, Photography, and the Crisis of the Union* (Baltimore: Johns Hopkins University Press, 1990).

7. Mary C. Gillett, *The Army Medical Department, 1818–1865* (Washington DC: U.S. Army Center of Military History, 1987), 275–86.

8. George Otis and Joseph J. Woodward, *Circular No. 6: Reports on the Extent and Nature of Materials . . . Medical and Surgical History of the Rebellion* (Washington DC: Government Printing Office, 1865), 2.

9. John Brinton, *Personal Memoirs of John H. Brinton* (New York: Neale Publishing Company, 1914), 186. While this initiative was not undertaken by Southern physicians, many specimens from Confederate soldiers who were treated at Union hospitals were shipped to Washington.

10. Robert S. Henry, *The Armed Forces Institute of Pathology: Its First Century, 1862–1962* (Washington DC: Office of the Surgeon General, 1964), 17–22.

11. *The Photographic Journal* 11 (1867), 205, quoted in Alison Gernsheim, "Medical Photography in the Nineteenth Century," *Medical and Biological Illustration* 11, no. 2 (1961): 85–92, 90.

12. William A. Hammond, *Circular No. 2* (1862), quoted in Henry, *The Armed Forces Institute*, 12.

13. Matthew Naythons, *The Face of Mercy: A Photographic History of Medicine at War* (New York: Random House, 1993), 61. The uses of these medical records are discussed in Robert Goler and Michael Rhode, "From Individual Trauma to National Policy: Tracking the Uses of Civil War Veteran Records," in *Disabled Veterans in History*, ed. David A. Gerber (Ann Arbor: University of Michigan Press, 2000), 163–84.

14. George Otis, *Surgical Photograph #93*, Army Medical Museum (Washington DC, 1865).

15. Alan Trachtenberg, *Reading American Photographs: Images as History* (New York: Hill and Wang, 1989), 116–8.

16. Geoffrey H. Hartman, "On Traumatic Knowledge and Literary Studies," *New Literary History* 26, no. 3 (1995) 537–63, 541n31.

17. Elaine Scarry, *The Body in Pain: The Making and Unmaking of the World* (New York: Oxford University Press, 1985), 63.

18. Gillett, *The Army Medical Department 1865–1917* (Washington DC: U.S. Army Center of Military History, 1995), 23; and Donald McMurry, "Pensions, Military and Naval," in *Dictionary of American History*, ed. James Truslow Adams (New York: Charles Scribner's Sons, 1940), 4:251.

19. For a summary of the political transformation of the pension system, particularly in the elections of 1884 and 1888, see Theda Skocpol, *Protecting Soldiers and Mothers: The Political Origins of Social Policy in the United States* (Cambridge: Harvard University Press, 1992), 120–30.

20. For an account of these changes, see Alan Green, "No Guts, No Glory," *Washington City Paper*, October 22, 1993, 24–31. Many of the amputee photographs and specimens remained at the Army Medical Museum (renamed the National Museum of Health and Medicine in 1989) and are available for scholarly research.

21. Trachtenberg, 118.

22. James T. H. Connor and Michael G. Rhode, "Shooting Soldiers: Civil War Medical Images, Memory, and Identity in America," *Invisible Culture: An Electronic Journal for Visual Culture* 5 (2002), http://www.rochester.edu/in_visible_culture/Issue_5/ConnorRhode/ConnorRhode.html (accessed March 30, 2004).

23. Sweet, 109.

24. Trachtenberg, 116. For a representative selection of these images, see Bradley P. Bengston and Julian E. Kuz, *Photographic Atlas of Civil War Injuries: Photographs of Surgical Cases and Specimens* (Grand Rapids, MI: Medical Staff Press, 1996). Some images also appear in Connor and Rhode, "Shooting Soldiers."

25. Cited in Goldner, 275.

26. This work was coauthored by two of Mitchell's colleagues. For a detailed account of Mitchell's experiences in this period, see William S. Middleton, "Turner's Lane Hospital," *Bulletin of the History of Medicine* 40 (1966): 14–42.

27. Debra Journet, "Phantom Limbs and 'Body-Ego': S. Weir Mitchell's 'George Dedlow,'" *Mosaic* 23 (Winter 1990): 87–99.

28. Mitchell's fictional, pseudo-scientific account appeared just months after the publication of Bernard's landmark methodological study, *Introduction à l'étude de la médicine expérimentale* (Paris: J. B. Baillière, 1865).

29. Mitchell, "The Medical Department," 1448.

30. Ibid., 1448–9.

31. Barbara Goldsmith, *Other Powers: The Age of Suffrage, Spiritualism, and the Scandalous Victoria Woodhull* (New York: Alfred A. Knopf, 1998), 28–37.

32. Guy Williams, *The Age of Miracles: Medicine and Surgery in the Nineteenth Century* (Chicago: Academy Press, 1987), 140–1. On the influence of electrotherapies on popular beliefs of individual vitality, see Harvey Green, *Fit for America: Health, Fitness, Sport, and American Society* (New York: Pantheon Books, 1986), 167–80.

33. Frederick L. M. Pattison, *Granville Sharp Pattison: Anatomist and Antagonist, 1791–1851* (Tuscaloosa: University of Alabama Press, 1987), 15.

34. Mitchell, "The Medical Department," 1449.

35. Lisa Herschbach, "'True Clinical Fictions': Medical and Literary Narratives from the Civil War Hospital," *Culture, Medicine, and Psychiatry* 19, no. 2 (1995): 183–205, 193 (Herschbach's italics).

36. Stanley S. Blair, "'A Dose of Exquisite Aesthetics': Literature in American Medicine, 1902–6," *Journal of Popular Culture* 28, no. 4 (1995): 103–12.

37. Herschbach, 199.

38. The *History* was issued in six volumes (Washington DC: Army Medical Museum, 1870–88). It is available as a reprint as United States Army Surgeon-General's Office, *The Medical and Surgical History of the Civil War*, 15 vols (Wilmington, NC: Broadfoot Publishing, 1990).

39. Connor and Rhode.

40. David E. Shi, *Facing Facts: Realism in American Thought and Culture, 1850–1920* (New York: Oxford University Press, 1995), 141–4; and Michael Fried, *Realism, Writing, Disfiguration on Thomas Eakins and Stephen Crane* (Chicago: University of Chicago Press, 1987), 5.

41. Fried, 61–2.

42. Goldner, 281.

43. Walt Whitman, "Death of President Lincoln," in *Specimen Days and Collect* (Philadelphia: Rees Welsh, 1882–83); available online at http://www.bartleby.com/229 (accessed March 30, 2004).

44. On charity and philanthropy in this period, see Robert H. Bremner, *The Public Good: Philanthropy and Welfare in the Civil War Era* (New York: Alfred A. Knopf, 1980), 144–78.

Extrapolating Race in *GATTACA*: Genetic Passing, Identity, and the Science of Race

David A. Kirby

Introduction

GATTACA (1997) is a rarity among science fiction films in that it transcended its mediocre box office earnings to become a common reference point in discussions about human-gene altering technologies.[1] As with *Brave New World*, another biologically based dystopian narrative, *GATTACA* provides a means of framing our relationships to new biotechnologies. News and magazine articles regularly use the phrase "GATTACA" when reporting discoveries in human genetics and biotechnology and their ethical implications. For example, the author of an article on reproductive medicine in *Wired* magazine wonders if allowing parents to select the gender of their offspring "would be a first step toward a *Gattaca*-like future of made-to-order babies, scrubbed clean of diseases and endowed with sparkling blue eyes—a world in which eugenics is just another branch of science."[2] Likewise, many television news programs highlight the ethical issues associated with human genetic engineering by showing clips of the film, such as CNN's *Newsroom*'s 2001 show about developments in genetic technologies.[3] In effect, these media outlets use the expression "GATTACA" to quickly conjure up images of a sterilized world where biotechnology has led to severe discrimination against the genetically unmodified. Educators also frequently use the film in a wide variety of classrooms, from junior high school through graduate school and from biology to English, to help teach about the bioethics of genetic technologies. One need only glance at the many online *GATTACA* teaching guides to see how the film has been widely acknowledged by educators as a text that conveys the ethical issues associated with human biotechnologies.[4]

Much of the science fiction cinema that extrapolates from emerging scientific theories and technologies explores socially troubling aspects of these new technologies. Following in this tradition, *GATTACA* projects from today's limited use of human biotechnologies to imagine a future where parents eagerly enhance the genetic makeup of their offspring. In this imagined future, limited access to genetic technologies sets up a two-tiered system of social organization: the genetically modified who represent the privileged, dominant group and the genetically unmodified who represent an oppressed group. During the course of the film the unmodified Vincent circumvents this genetic discrimination by passing off the genes of the enhanced Eugene as his own. In a previous essay, I demonstrated that *GATTACA* works as a successful bioethical text because it does not fault human genetic technologies.[5] Rather, the film warns that these technologies will create problems only if society accepts a genetic determinist ideology that sees humans as nothing more than the sum of their genes.

GATTACA extrapolates not only from current technological trajectories but also from current ideological trajectories in that it projects a world of total genetic determinism from today's movement toward "geneticization." Geneticization, a phrase coined by geneticist Abby Lippman, describes the trend in American society toward a reductionist view of humanity as a collection of genes. As Lippman defines it, "Geneticization refers to an ongoing process by which differences between individuals are reduced to their DNA codes, with most disorders, behaviors and physiological variations defined, at least in part, as genetic in origin."[6] *GATTACA* shows the ultimate consequence of this trend: a world where a person's only sense of identity comes from his or her genes.

Although *GATTACA* succeeds in its social criticism of genetic determinism, its extrapolation of a eugenic world from trends in geneticization ignores the equally problematic contemporary trend toward the scientific linking of genes and racial differences. The film's discussion of genetic determinism and eugenics does not take into account current attempts by social conservatives to define race genetically, or the role race has played in the history of eugenics. Although *GATTACA* relies on the recognizable tropes of racial discrimination to support its claims about genetic discrimination, it ignores contemporary issues of race and genetics in America. In actuality, *GATTACA* functions as a "passing" film that utilizes terminology, images, and situations familiar in discussions of racial discrimination.

Methodologies and Interpretive Framework

In his studies of race and *Star Trek*, Daniel Bernardi applies neo-Marxist theory to this example of extrapolative science fiction in order to critique the understanding of the current hegemonic structure it suggests. According to Bernardi, knowledge of past culture is essential for understanding the trajectory from past hegemony to the present hegemonic structure. Therefore, we cannot overlook the historical significance of race when examining present-day hegemony. Likewise, if we wish to plot an extrapolative trajectory into the future we cannot overlook contemporary hegemony. Thus, he interprets *Star Trek: The Next Generation* as a neoconservative projection from contemporary society to a "white future-time" open to all minorities and aliens who are willing to be assimilated to this ostensibly progressive society. Bernardi argues that we define "progressive" society based on a white American norm. The Trek universe, specifically the "United Federation of Planets," is the cultural inheritor of American societal goals and ideals. Multiculturalism, as a Trek/American ideal, is represented by the *Enterprise*'s heterogeneous crew including the dark-skinned alien Klingons, but it is embedded within assumptions that races/species conform within Federation/white American standards.[7] The utopian vision of race in the future society extrapolated by *GATTACA*, however, begs the question of how the filmmakers envision a racially harmonious future based on the contemporary state of racial division and discrimination in America, which does not envision new racial relationships.

According to Antonio Gramsci, the ruling class, in order to maintain its hegemonic position, must legitimate and renew the "common sense" mentality in society through consent or coercion. Scientific validation is a powerful mode for generating consent because it makes the prevailing common sense seem inevitable, i.e., "the natural order of things." Gramsci recognized this relationship between science and consent. In the *Prison Notebooks*, he writes, "Philosophy and modern science are constantly contributing new elements to 'modern folklore' [common sense] in that certain opinions and scientific notions, removed from their context and more or less distorted, constantly fall within the popular domain and are 'inserted' into the mosaic of tradition."[8] Gramsci's notion of the "insertion" of scientific elements into the "mosaic of tradition" is comparable to the science and technology studies concept of "black boxing," which refers to scientific theories that society accepts as being accurate and useful descriptions of nature. Bruno Latour provides a theoretical framework for understanding the role that mass media, like fictional films, can play in the establishment of scientific black boxes.[9] Latour maintains that scientific concepts become black boxed when the concept has a significant number of "allies" who are convinced that it represents an accurate portrayal of nature. Once a scientific concept is black boxed, it is thought of as "common sense" and the ruling class can use it to legitimate its dominance. Allies for a scientific concept can come from any segment of society, including popular cultural forms like fictional films. In Latour's theoretical framework, science fiction films like GATTACA can play a significant role in the social acceptance of scientific concepts.

GATTACA as a "Passing" Film

Several filmic elements in GATTACA show a clear analogy between the genetic discrimination faced by genetically unmodified people and racial discrimination faced by minorities in contemporary American society. First, the terminology surrounding genetic discrimination in the film conjures up words associated with contemporary racial discrimination. For example, Vincent, in one of his voice-overs, explains, "It's illegal to discriminate on the basis of genetics—genoism it's called—but no one takes the laws seriously." The voice-over is delivered in a flashback in which Vincent is waiting to interview for a job that he knows he will never get because of his genetic makeup. As with racism in contemporary America, genoism may be illegal, but it is clearly practiced in the society portrayed by GATTACA. Likewise, just as minorities are often referred to by derogatory names, so too are the genetically unmodified referred to by disparaging names, such as "faith births," "defectives," "God children," or the officially sanctioned term "in-valids." In-valids who utilize the genetics of the genetically modified are called "de-gene-erates" or "borrowed ladders."

Vincent experiences all the obstacles that a minority might experience in present-day American society: joblessness, lack of educational opportunities, alienation, low self-esteem, etc. Like a dark-skinned individual whose minority status is visible to all, Vincent's position as genetically unmodified, albeit invisible, is easily ascertained. Vincent explains in the flashback that anything he touches, a door handle, a handshake, or the saliva on a letter, could provide a sample of his DNA and identify him as a genetically unmodified individual. Furthermore, his minority status, as with many minorities today, prevents him from getting jobs for which he would otherwise be eligible. Although his genes prevent him from obtaining a formal education, Vincent manages to educate himself as an engineer. In the flashback, Vincent, in a voice-over, informs us that, in hindsight, he should have known he would never be hired for an engineering job: "It didn't matter how much I lied on my resume. My real resume was in my cells." Since poor vision is an indication that an individual is not modified, he removes his glasses before the interview. As he opens the door, a series of close-ups accompanied by his voice-over underscores the fact that removing his glasses was futile: the company could easily obtain a DNA sample, and thus his identity. Realizing that the company will not hire him because of his minority status, he leaves before the interview even starts.

In several scenes, socially imposed obstacles are made literal in order to illustrate discrimination against unmodified individuals. For example, a scene in which a teacher informs Vincent's parents that he cannot go to school with other children ends with a close-up of a gate closing on Vincent. The visual composition of the scene emphasizes that Vincent's genetic makeup "closes the door" on his educational opportunities. In another scene, the "glass ceiling" that exists when discrimination is illegal but openly practiced is literally depicted. Vincent is shown working as a janitor at the Gattaca Corporation, with his face pressed against a glass window, looking at the genetically modified individuals who work inside.

Vincent eventually obtains an engineering job at Gattaca by procuring modified DNA that he passes off as his own. He seeks out a DNA broker, German, who specializes in finding valids willing to "rent out" their genetic material to in-valids. German matches Vincent with Eugene, a former Olympic swimmer who lost the use of his legs after a failed suicide attempt.[10] In exchange, Eugene receives a portion of Vincent's salary. To succeed at the deception, Eugene collects his body material—hair, skin cells, eyelashes, urine, and blood—for Vincent to use when he is subjected to rigorous genetic measurements. Likewise, Vincent must vigorously scrub himself to remove loose skin and hair that could betray his true identity.

By borrowing Eugene's "good genes" or "DNA ladder," Vincent is comparable to minority characters in other films who avoid discrimination and obtain jobs by passing as a member of the majority group. For example, in the film *Lost Boundaries* (1949), an African American doctor passes as white in order to get a better job at a prestigious hospital. Other, more recent examples of films that depict passing to gain economic advantage include *School Ties* (1992), *Devil in a Blue Dress* (1995), and the British film *Skin Deep* (2001). The comedy *The Associate* (1996) even took the concept of passing to the extreme of having an

African American female pass as a white male in order to succeed in business. In his book *Neither Black Nor White Yet Both*, Werner Sollors claims that a "significant number of cases of 'passing'" occur only in situations of "sharp inequality between groups."[11] Such is the case in *GATTACA*. Moreover, the boundary that separates the two groups can easily be assessed: the Gattaca Corporation maintains entrance stations to validate a person's genetic identity and turn away in-valids. Even average citizens can obtain other people's genetic information. For example, Vincent's love interest, Irene, has his (really Eugene's) DNA analyzed at a "sequencing" station. The many close-ups of Vincent's body matter (hair, skin, blood, etc.) show the risk he faces that anyone could easily determine his true identity. Ultimately, Vincent's eyelash found near a crime scene points to him as a murderer, at least in the minds of the police. Given that every cell contains genetic information, the ability to pass as one of the genetically modified becomes exceed-ingly difficult. What makes *GATTACA* unique as a passing film is that Vincent, a white male, is passing as another white male whose differ-ences are invisible to the naked eye but easily detectable in the genetically obsessed future society.

Like many other minorities who wish to pass, the genetically unmodified Vincent will do anything in order to overcome discrimina-tion, including undertaking extreme physical changes. The extent to which Vincent is willing to alter his physical appearance is reminiscent of procedures historically used by some African Americans in order to make them appear white. These procedures included the use of bleach-ing agents to remove melanin and lighten the skin and the use of strong detergents, such as lye, to denature kinky hair. A scene from *Malcolm X* (1992) when Red/Malcolm X is unable to wash out a straightening chemical and burns his scalp demonstrates just how painful these processes could be. In *GATTACA*, one scene gruesomely illustrates the lengths to which Vincent will go in order to join the ranks of the genetically modified. After some minor physical alterations, German informs Vincent that he is not tall enough to pass for Eugene. Vincent's response ("Can't I just wear lifts?") is met with a knowing glance between German and Eugene. Vincent realizes what they have in mind and protests that he will not do "that." Eugene, who is relying on Vincent's potential income to support his standard of living, questions Vincent's desire to follow through on their arrangement: "I thought you were serious, Vincent?" A quick cut to a radial bone saw follows Vincent's response, and we realize that Vincent is having his legs extended. The scene then fades to a shot of Vincent lying on the ground with his legs in braces. Vincent's voice-over tells us that Eugene "never questioned my commitment again." That Vincent is willing to undertake such a painful procedure demonstrates the lengths he is willing to go to pass as a member of the dominant group.[12]

Genetic passing performs two functions in GATTACA. First, as discussed above, the filmmakers use the concept of passing as a means for furthering the analogy between racial discrimination and genetic discrimination. The second function of passing in GATTACA is to call into question the origins and maintenance of the identity categories and boundaries set up by genetic determinism. Within the world imagined by GATTACA, the dominant class's grounds of privilege are founded upon the complete acceptance of genetic determinism. In Passing and the Fictions of Identity, Elaine K. Ginsberg argues that the act of passing destabilizes grounds of privilege that are founded on essentialism.[13] Genetic determinism is the ultimate essentialist ideology because it claims human beings are nothing more than the sum of their genes. Therefore, GATTACA forces us to ask this question: If the genetically unmodified can pass as genetically modified, then what is genetic modification actually accomplishing? Since the genetically unmodified Vincent passes as a modified individual and proves to be more successful than all the modified characters, GATTACA undermines the very basis of genetic discrimination and the boundary between unmodified and modified.

Getting From Here to There: The Extrapolation of Racial (In)Equality in GATTACA

To adopt Gramsci's terms, the genetically modified in GATTACA are the dominant class who legitimate their hegemonic position through fostering a total belief in the genetic determinist ideology. The idea that determination of self is solely based on genetic makeup is seen as "common sense" and is taken as the "natural" order of things in this future society. One way to ascertain the dominant class is by identifying the group which other groups must pass as in order to gain economic advantage (opportunistic passing). In GATTACA, it is clear that the genetically modified are the dominant group since the unmodified Vincent can only gain economic advantage by passing as a modified individual. According to Ginsberg, the discourse of passing in American history has been predicated upon the assumption that white males occupy a place of status and privilege in society.[14] Passing stories where minority men or white women pass as white males to gain economic

advantage show us not only that minorities and women occupy peripheral groups but that white males are the dominant class. But in
GATTACA it is a white male who has to pass in order to obtain the
privileges of the dominant class. Ginsberg's assumption about privileged white male status is not valid in this extrapolated future society
in which white males per se no longer occupy the dominant class. By
setting up a white male as the character who must pass as a member
of a ruling class (Eugene is also white; his genetic modification gives
him his status), GATTACA sets up an extrapolated hegemony that is
contrary to the current white hegemony.

Outside of the fact that a white male must pass to join the
privileged class, there are other elements from the film that suggest that
race no longer forms a barrier separating people in this society. The film
takes the "Star Trek" view of race in the future, in that there are many
minority characters whose race plays no significance.[15] This vision of
racial blindness is reminiscent of what Micheal Pounds calls the "United
Nations" version of the future as seen in Star Trek.[16] Pounds says that
as "American society struggles with redefining the workplace as inclu-
sive of the nation's diversity, both Star Trek series modeled a workplace
where men and women, whites and blacks, and aliens functioned
together as professional equals."[17] Several minority characters have
positions of power in GATTACA. Both the geneticist who helps Vincent's
parents design a second child and the first person to interview Vincent
are African Americans. These characters are designed to present a "race-
blind" society in which the only concern is genetics and not skin color
or ethnicity. Every shot of the workers inside the Gattaca Corporation
shows a mix of races and ethnicities, men and women. In addition,
every scene inside the nightclub/restaurant frequented by the genetically modified includes an ethnically diverse group of people. Likewise,
the only other group of genetically modified workers we see, the police,
includes several African Americans. At Vincent's first interview, the
waiting room shows a wide mix of races and genders, with the
implication that all of these people have a shot at this job—the
exception being Vincent, whose glasses give him away as a member of
the only minority class in this future world. On the other side of the
genetic barrier, the only in-valids who are shown in the film are white
males. In fact, every in-valid shown in the film is a white male. This
includes all the in-valids rounded up in the murder investigation and
all the janitors who clean the Gattaca Corporation.

One scene is particularly useful in illustrating the filmmakers'
attempt to present a "Star Trek" future of racial equality. After Vincent

has boarded a rocket near the end of the film there is a shot of the other engineers accompanying him into space. The camera starts in on a close-up of an African American male's face, then the camera pans from right to left, revealing an Asian male, a white male, an Asian woman, and finally resting on Vincent's face. According to the dominant ideology of this society, the only individual who should not be on this rocket is the genetically unmodified white male, Vincent. Like *Star Trek*, *GATTACA* offers a utopian vision of a multicultural workplace where job discrimination based on race and gender is a thing of the past. Individuals from any ethnic group can get a job at the prestigious Gattaca Corporation, as long as they have the proper genetic makeup.

This utopian vision of a postracist society flows from the assumption that an individual's identity emerges only from his or her genetic makeup. If society defines you solely on the basis of your genes, then there is no longer any need for associations grounded on other factors. In *GATTACA*, cultural groups are seemingly no longer socially constructed but, rather, are biologically constructed. Associations based on genetics are so strong, in fact, that genetic allegiance overrides familial identity. In "The New Eugenics in Cinema," I demonstrated how the depictions of blood in *GATTACA* serve as metaphors for genetic identity.[18] Blood as a metaphor for individual genetic identity even transcends the use of blood to define familial relationships: Vincent's genetically modified brother, Anton, declines Vincent's attempt to become his "blood brother." Anton's rejection of Vincent's "defective" blood indicates his preference for relationships based on the quality of an individual's genes rather than on larger bonds of kinship. Given the rejection of familial associations in favor of genetic associations, it is not surprising that other cultural relationships break down in *GATTACA's* genetic determinist society.

In essence, *GATTACA* sets up a dystopian world in regard to genes and a utopian world in regard to race. This utopian vision of a race-blind society in *GATTACA*, however, is not extrapolated from the state of racial division and discrimination in American society today. At the risk of oversimplification, there are two opposing views on how to define race, the biological and the sociological. The biological definition assumes that races are different in physical, mental, and behavioral characteristics that reflect significant underlying genetic differentiation. The sociological definition, on the other hand, assumes that race is socially constructed from shared historical relationships and experiences. Given that the film ultimately attacks any notion that genes can truly define people, it is not surprising that the filmmakers adopt a social constructionist view of race. However, by ignoring the possibility that the biological definition of race could become "common sense," the filmmakers overlook another danger arising from unlimited uses of human genetic technologies.

Contemporary Scientific Racism and the Extrapolation of Race in *GATTACA*

The racially harmonious society portrayed in *GATTACA* does not project today's social conservativism, which extends genetic determinism to include a biological definition of race. By defining race genetically, social conservatives link behavioral and intellectual differences to underlying genetic differences. Moreover, throughout its history, eugenics has been intricately linked to the genetic definition of race.[19] Most proponents of a "new," technologically driven eugenics argue that we are beyond the "historical mistakes" of the old eugenics and its racial baggage. Ashley Montagu contends that this view is misguided because "the dead hand of the past may continue to guide the practice of the present as well of the future."[20] Steven Selden also sounds a warning in his book on race and eugenics, noting that "such ignorance of the past is potentially dangerous."[21]

It is not difficult to find recent examples of behavioral geneticists and "evolutionary psychologists" who claim to have found genetic differences among races that account for mental or behavioral traits. Perhaps the best-known examples are Richard Herrnstein and Charles Murray, who in their 1994 bestseller, *The Bell Curve*, claim that disparities in IQ scores among Asians, whites, and Africans are due to underlying genetic differences.[22] Although intelligence may be the best-known trait for current researchers who wish to link race and genetics, it is certainly not the only one. Behaviors, such as violence and criminality, and personality characteristics, such as "childhood shyness," are also traits for which researchers claim to have found genetic links and significant differences among races.[23] Other work that has received recent publicity relates to the supposed genetic basis for African Americans' prowess in athletics as promoted by Jon Entine in *Taboo: Why Black Athletes Dominate Sports and Why We're Afraid to Talk about It*.[24]

Developmental psychologist Richard Lynn sees the growing list of genetic differences among races as a sign that a new eugenics is *desirable*. In his 2001 book, *Eugenics: A Reassessment*, Lynn makes the case that at the end of the twentieth century "a wide measure of consensus had already been reached" in regard to "the genetic contri-

bution . . . to intelligence, and to personality." Because of "the importance of intelligence and personality for educational and occupational
achievement," Lynn believes that equality will only be reached by using
our burgeoning new biotechnologies. Of course, in Lynn's view some
racial groups have more of an uphill genetic battle than others. He cites
The Bell Curve as a "portent of the coming counterrevolution in the
rehabilitation of eugenics."[25] Few geneticists, however, go as far as
Lynn. Most behavioral geneticists and evolutionary psychologists who
advocate racial differences based on genetics claim that they are only
revealing "nature as it is." It should not come as a surprise, however,
that these supposed differences favor current white power structures.

   According to biologists Richard Lewontin, Steven Rose, and Leon
Kamin, genetic determinism has been "a powerful mode of explaining
the observed inequalities of status, wealth, and power in contemporary
industrial capitalist societies." They sound a warning in their book, *Not
in Our Genes*, that neoconservatives, who Lewontin et al. call the New
Right, have increasingly turned to genetic determinism and biological
definitions of race to justify their privileged position. Lewontin et al.
contend that genetic determinism "has been gratefully seized upon as
a political legitimator by the New Right, which finds its social nostrums
so neatly mirrored in nature; for if these inequalities are biologically
determined, they are therefore inevitable and immutable." [26] Lewontin
et al. are not alone in interpreting the New Right's attempts to define
racial differences genetically as efforts to legitimate the current power
structure as "natural." Ruth Hubbard and Elijah Wald link the rise in
behavioral genetics to a conservative political climate:

> This shift is due in part to a conservative backlash against the gains
> of the civil rights and women's rights movements. These and similar
> movements have emphasized the importance of our environment in
> shaping who we are, insisting that women, African Americans, and
> other kinds of people have an inferior status in American society
> because of prejudices against them, not because of any natural
> inferiority. Conservatives are quick to hail scientific discoveries that
> seem to show innate differences which they can use to explain the
> current social order.[27]

Biologist Stephen Jay Gould also perceives *The Bell Curve* as just another
attempt to make racial inequalities a "natural" outcome of "inherent"
differences in intelligence. According to Gould, "The remarkable impact
of *The Bell Curve* must therefore, and once again as always, be recording

a swing of the political pendulum to a sad position that requires a rationale for affirming social inequalities as dictates of biology."[28]

Those wanting to challenge racial social policies, especially affirmative action, have certainly seized upon *The Bell Curve*'s findings. For example, Thomas Sowell, a senior fellow at the conservative Hoover Institution, wrote an article for *American Spectator* in which he states, "In thus demolishing the foundation underlying such practices as double-standards in college admissions and 'race-norming' of employment tests, *The Bell Curve* threatens both a whole generation of social policies and the careers of those who promote them."[29] Likewise, in an article for *National Review*, Michael Barone wrote:

> More specifically, by showing strong relationships between intelligence as measured by IQ tests and behaviors ranging from job performance to a propensity to commit crimes or bear children outside marriage, *The Bell Curve* makes a powerful case that the disproportionately low number of blacks in top positions and the disproportionately high number of blacks in prison (just under half our prisoners are black) do not result from racial discrimination.[30]

More worryingly, books such as *The Bell Curve* enable eugenic ideas to get a hearing among the "respectable" right. A review in *American Spectator* warned about "the worsening of the American gene pool" and even raised the question of criminal sterilization as a possible solution.[31] While *The Bell Curve* received the most response from the general press, it is not the only mainstream book to make such claims or to tie them to social policies. Conservatives have seized upon other books, such as J. Philippe Rushton's *Race, Evolution, and Behavior* and Michael Levin's *Why Race Matters*, as "scientific proof" of genetic racial differences and evidence that affirmative-action policies are "unnatural."[32]

Hubbard, Wald, and other critics of scientific racism point out that efforts to justify racial differences based on genetics are not new. Their concern, however, is that current attempts to find genetic differences among races come at a time when the American public is more and more convinced that genetic technologies are revealing the natural "truth" about humanity. From the perspective of scientific racism's critics, the move to make genetic determinism "common sense" can never be independent from scientific attempts to correlate race and genetics. In light of this association between genetic determinism and race in the history of American eugenics, it is surprising that *GATTACA*'s filmmakers failed to take into account contemporary arguments by neoconservatives linking race and genetics.

GATTACA's failure to address race and genetics is unfortunate, because popular films play a significant role in the acceptance or rejection of certain scientific ideas. Proponents of a genetic basis for race claim that the establishment of genetic racial differences is inevitable because "nature" has the final say. As is the case with all knowledge production, the establishment of scientific facts requires social acceptance, and this acceptance requires interactions among various actors. The diffusion of genetic explanations to all aspects of society is not an obvious consequence of scientific advancement but the result of complex interactions and negotiations. Therefore, the production of "scientific fact" is at stake in any attempts to translate genetic claims to the general public.

Black boxing can occur without the endorsement of the scientific community if a critical mass of the public accepts the concept as "representing reality." Despite the urging of molecular biologists that genetic explanations must take into account environmental factors, fringe sociologists have employed behavioral genetics and evolutionary psychology to establish a prominent public discourse about genetics. Critiquing such approaches, Dorothy Nelkin and Susan Lindee have shown how the gene has become a cultural icon and how genetic determinist notions permeate popular culture.[33] Peter Conrad's work demonstrates how the news media fail to report disconfirmations and often misrepresent genetic findings by adopting a frame of "genetic optimism" that has led to a privileging of genetics in public discourse.[34] José Van Dijck shows how, in the mass media, the genetic frame has become common for explaining a wider range of societal problems.[35] In essence, these sociological studies demonstrate the black boxing of genetic determinism over the objections of molecular biologists. GATTACA is a popular culture exception that does not serve as an ally for genetic determinism. Regrettably, while it presents a strong statement against the black boxing of a genetic determinist ideology, it misses an equally important opportunity to keep the black box of genetic racial differences from closing.

Conclusion

That we are headed for a "new" eugenics is clear. The near completion of the Human Genome Project was announced in spring of 2001 with the publication of 99 percent of a human's DNA sequence.[36]

Although this information will have limited use initially, in the not-too-distant future humans will soon be able to use this knowledge in conjunction with new genetic technologies to determine the genetic makeup of offspring before they are born. Recent major developments in human genetic technologies have made the likelihood of wholesale genetic changes even greater and have moved us one step closer to a GATTACA-like future. For example, in several cases, reproductive technicians used preimplantation embryonic selection, the technology used in GATTACA, to select embryos that did not contain known genetic defects. In one highly publicized case, a couple was able to select an embryo that did not carry the allele for Fanconi's anemia (a blood disease) before implantation in the mother's womb.[37] There have also been some successes in germ-line gene therapy with our close relative the rhesus monkey.[38] According to an article in Wired magazine, these developments render the question of a new eugenics irrelevant: "The fact is, eugenics is here. Brought to you by high technology and the free market, it looks nothing like a Nazi newsreel. The question isn't 'Should we have eugenics?' but rather, 'How far should we go?'"[39] Unfortunately, the ethical question of "How far should we go?" is too simplistic. There are many other ethical problems embedded within the new eugenics. As I have argued in this essay, two scientific ideologies will have a profound impact on the direction the new eugenics will take if they become black boxed: genetic determinism and a genetic definition of race.

Fictional films, like GATTACA, will play a role in determining whether these scientific ideologies become black boxed. Rather than serving as another popular culture ally for genetic determinism, GATTACA provides a powerful counterexample. However, the society envisioned within GATTACA in which racial inequality no longer exists is not only overly optimistic but ignores an alarming, persistent racial ideology that seeks to define some races as genetically inferior. This omission undercuts the film's perceptive critique of genetic determinism because it offers minority viewers the vision that enhanced genetics can lead to the path of racial equality. By presenting a raceless society obsessed with genetics, the film suggests that genetic determinism combined with genetic manipulation will have some desirable consequences. In this genetically deterministic world, equality is not achieved through complex social changes but through the simplistic route of genetic manipulation. As Nelkin and Lindee demonstrate, genetic explanations have a powerful appeal because they offer simple solutions and displace blame for social problems from external, societal causes to internal, biological causes. For social conservatives, a genetic basis for racial differences provides easy answers and justification for current inequalities and discrimination. According to this viewpoint, unrestricted manipulation of human genetics would be a good thing because it would allow "inferior races" to remove these "defective elements" and would lead to racial equality, as shown in *GATTACA*. This simplistic and racist viewpoint rests upon the belief that people will have equal access to gene-altering technologies, should such a future presents itself. Social inequality often leads to unequal access to scientific benefits, and a consensus that race has an underlying genetic basis would actually accelerate social problems. The black boxing of a genetic basis for race would provide scientific justification for current discriminatory practices and deepen the racial and ethnic income gap. Rather than leading to the racial utopia as depicted in *GATTACA*, the acceptance of a genetic basis of race will only further segregate society.

NOTES

1. *GATTACA*, directed by Andrew Niccol, 1997, Columbia Tristar Pictures. The title of the film is actually an acronym of sorts. The letters G-A-T-T-A-C-A refer to the four DNA bases, adenosine, guanosine, thymine, and cytosine. Therefore the title of the movie, *GATTACA*, mimics a DNA sequence.

2. Brendan I. Koerner, "Embryo Police," *Wired* 10, no. 2 (2002): 53.

3. Joel Hochmuth, "Voyage of Life," *CNN Newsroom*, May 3, 2001. Transcript of the show can be found at http://www.cnn.com/TRANSCRIPTS/0105/03/nr.00.html (accessed March 19, 2004).

4. For example, see http://www.teachwithmovies.org/guides/Gattaca.html (accessed March 19, 2004).

5. David A. Kirby, "The New Eugenics in Cinema: Genetic Determinism and Gene Therapy in *GATTACA*," *Science Fiction Studies* 27, no. 2 (2000): 193–215.

6. Abby Lippman, "Prenatal Genetic Testing and Screening: Constructing Needs and Reinforcing Inequities," *American Journal of Law and Medicine* 17 (1991): 15–50, 19.

7. Daniel Bernardi, *Star Trek and History: Race-ing Toward a White Future* (New Brunswick, NJ: Rutgers University Press, 1998), 135–6.

8. Antonio Gramsci, *Selections from Cultural Writings*, ed. Geoffrey Nowell Smith and trans. William Boelhower (Cambridge: Harvard University Press, 1985), 189.

9. Bruno Latour, *Science in Action: How to Follow Scientists and Engineers through Society* (Cambridge: Harvard University Press, 1987).

10. Eugene's full name is Eugene Morrow, which suggests the "good gene of tomorrow" and thus refers to eugenics.

11. Werner Sollors, *Neither Black Nor White Yet Both* (New York: Oxford University Press, 1997), 248.

12. This is not to say that white men are not members of the dominant group (e.g., Eugene) or that white men exclusively occupy fringe status in the society extrapolated by *GATTACA*. Rather, genetics, not skin color, determines one's inclusion in the privileged class.

13. Elaine K. Ginsberg, "Introduction: The Politics of Passing," in *Passing and the Fictions of Identity*, ed. Elaine K. Ginsberg (Durham, NC: Duke University Press, 1996), 1–16.

14. Ibid.

15. The "Star Trek" view of a racially harmonious future world is discussed in Bernardi, *Star Trek and History*; Jon Wagner and Jan Lundeen, *Deep Space and Sacred Time* (Westport, CT: Praeger, 1998); and Micheal Pounds, *Race in Space* (Lanham, MD: Scarecrow Press, 1999).

16. Pounds, 52.

17. Ibid., 91.

18. Kirby, 206–7.

19. For the history of eugenics and its racial dimensions see Donald K. Pickens, *Eugenics and the Progressives* (Nashville: Vanderbilt University Press, 1968); Daniel J. Kevles, *In the Name of Eugenics* (New York: Alfred A. Knopf, 1985); Marouf A. Hasian, *The Rhetoric of Eugenics in Anglo-American Thought* (Athens: University of Georgia Press, 1996); and Steven Selden, *Inheriting Shame: The Story of Eugenics and Racism in America* (New York: Teachers College Press, 1999).

20. Montagu's quote is found in his foreword to Selden, *Inheriting Shame*, vii.

21. Ibid., xv.

22. Richard J. Herrnstein and Charles Murray, *The Bell Curve: Intelligence and Class Structure in American Life* (New York: Free Press, 1994).

23. Summaries of research in behavioral genetics can be found in William Wright, *Born That Way: Genes, Behavior, Personality* (New York: Alfred A. Knopf, 1998).

24. Jon Entine, *Taboo: Why Black Athletes Dominate Sports and Why We're Afraid to Talk about It* (New York: Public Affairs, 2000).

25. Richard Lynn, *Eugenics: A Reassessment* (Westport, CT: Praeger, 2001), 275.

26. Richard C. Lewontin, Steven Rose, and Leon J. Kamin, *Not in Our Genes* (New York: Pantheon Books, 1984), 7.

27. Ruth Hubbard and Elijah Wald, *Exploding the Gene Myth* (Boston: Beacon Press, 1997), 9. The view that social conservatives are the only ones supporting a genetic definition of race is too simplistic. For example, Marouf Hasian's research shows the ways in which some African Americans have supported eugenics. Hasian, *The Rhetoric of Eugenics*, 51–71.

28. Stephen Jay Gould, *The Mismeasure of Man* (New York: W. W. Norton, 1996), 31.

29. Thomas Sowell, "Ethnicity and IQ," *American Spectator* 28, no. 1 (1995): 32–6, 32.

30. Michael Barone, "Common Knowledge," *National Review* 46, no. 23 (1994): 32–4, 34.

31. Christopher Caldwell, review of *The Bell Curve*, by Richard J. Herrnstein and Charles Murray, *American Spectator* 28, no. 1 (1995): 62–7, 67.

32. J. Philippe Rushton, *Race, Evolution, and Behavior* (New Brunswick, NJ: Transaction, 1995); and Michael E. Levin, *Why Race Matters*, (Westport, CT: Prager, 1997).

33. Dorothy Nelkin and M. Susan Lindee, *The DNA Mystique: The Gene as a Cultural Icon* (New York: W. H. Freeman, 1995).

34. Peter Conrad, "Public Eyes and Private Genes: Historical Frames, News Constructions, and Social Problems," *Social Problems* 44, no. 2 (1997): 139–54; and Peter Conrad and Dana Weinberg, "Has the Gene for Alcoholism Been Discovered Three Times since 1980?" *Perspectives on Social Problems* 8 (1996): 3–24.

35. José Van Dijck, *Imagenation: Popular Images of Genetics* (New York: New York University Press, 1998).

36. Rick Weiss, "Life's Blueprint in Less Than an Inch," *Washington Post*, February 11, 2001, A1.

    37. Peter Gorner, "Embryo is Picked to Try to Save Sister's Life," *Chicago Tribune*, October 2, 2000, 1.
    38. Rick Weiss, "Scientists Create First Genetically Altered Monkey," *Washington Post*, January 12, 2001, A1.
    39. Brian Alexander, "The Remastered Race," *Wired* 10, no. 5 (2002): 68.

Response to Section III: Dis-embodiment

Joel Howell

This trio of essays treats the reader to three seemingly distinct yet fundamentally complementary visions of how to think about human health and disease. Stephen Rachman tells us about the tightly bounded (both geographically and conceptually) worlds of the Cantonese artist Lam Qua and the American medical missionary Peter Parker in early nineteenth-century Canton. Robert Goler unpacks the imagined world of "The Case of George Dedlow," a quadruple amputee from the American War between the States who was created in 1866 by the young (and soon to be famous) Philadelphia physician S. Weir Mitchell. David Kirby critiques how the 1997 science fiction movie *GATTACA* addresses contemporary ideas about eugenics, race, and society in a futuristic world where a person of any skin color or racial/ethnic background can get a good job, as long as he or she has the right genetic makeup.

These three essays carry us from distant past to distant future, from worlds of distorted and absent body parts to worlds of idealized and perfect body parts. Each world utilizes the latest and best science and technology of the day to create and track the illusion of progress or perfection. Although distant in time and space, these worlds were created with the facade of verisimilitude that masks the fact that they do not exist outside of the creator's mind. In their critiques of these worlds, all three essays remind us of the power of art to re-create beauty as well as to make us cringe from the horror of unspeakable wounds. They allow the reader to witness vicariously the medical messiness of these unpleasant, disordered worlds and force us to reexamine our notion of archetype.

I will focus on how these essays deal with the tension between generalizability and specificity, on the one hand, and theory and practice, on the other, on how they reflect the tension between lofty ideals and the inherent messiness of life, of medicine, and of health care. Health-care workers today are acutely aware of the metaphorical and literal messiness of the medical world, that variability is part of physicians' professional socialization. Each year I teach a class in law and medicine to law and medical students. Far more important than the differences in content and knowledge that the students of these two professions bring to the class is the difference in their approach. For example, when faced with a dilemma such as "How should we manage treatment at the end of life?" law students are prone to give theoretically rich yet practically unusable answers. After considerable reading and contemplation, they often produce a simple answer: "When medical therapy is futile, you should stop." They then close their hands and sit back, confident that they have produced an effective solution for the problem at hand. Medical students, on the other hand, having drunk deeply from the well of individuality, have come to expect and to revel in medical messiness, and, despite a solid grounding in any number of relevant disciplines, if asked to describe their general approach to a patient will often say quite sincerely, "There is no general approach. Each patient is unique." Indeed so, but if a physician (or a physician-in-training) truly started at first principles each time she or he entered the examining room, each encounter would take a long, long time! That tension between the theoretical and the applied, the archetypal model and the infinitely variable person, the tidy ideal and the messy reality of human existence is part of the underlying theme for each of the essays in this section.

Lam Qua's dramatic paintings of Parker's patients give us the possibility of idealized perfection, portraying figures who will never succumb to their disease; they are frozen in time and space. Yet at the same time he was making these medical images, Lam Qua was producing vast quantities of standardized images in a factory-like system. That he participated in such mass production was used as evidence that he was not a true "artist" in the fanciful, idealized sense. By being able to produce repetitive images for sale, Lam Qua both displayed great skill and exhibited a trait thought to contradict artistry. Parker, too, was running a busy clinical system, seeing hundreds of patients a day by using a form of labor-intensive mass production. Both Parker and Lam Qua gained skill through repetition, skill that helped each to better achieve his goals. While some of his paintings may have been mass produced, the individuality of Lam Qua's medical images emphasizes the specific nature of each patient, each tumor, the idea that medicine proceeds one by one, case by case, individual by individual. Parker praised the quality of both the "likeness" of the person and the "representation" of the disease state.

In "The Case of George Dedlow," standardization is key to the story. The removed limbs have not simply been left on the battlefield for the vultures; they have been taken back to a central repository, the Army Medical Museum, not simply to sit and rot (although the partial decomposition from being stored in a vat of alcohol of the specific limbs in question [3486 & 3487] makes them unable to bear for long the weight of the imagined apparition) but to be counted, categorized, and studied. In this world, casualties are also made visible through the new technology of photography. In an age in which soldiers who lost a limb had done so without benefit of anesthesia, either on the battlefield or through a frenzied two-minute amputation shortly thereafter (if fortunate enough to have the procedure done by a skilled surgeon), the mental wounds were no doubt quite real, yet "Dedlow" chose to portray visible wounds rather than invisible mental anguish. This approach to documentation was part of an effort to make nineteenth-century America a rationalized, structured modern world. The counting served to reify the horrendous toll of war: the almost inconceivable numbers of casualties made visible through scientific record keeping, through measuring and labeling, and through counting and categorizing. The individual gained stature by being part of a larger, organized group.

In GATTACA, standardization is also the fundamental underpinning of the story. The very title of the film evokes the ultimate standardization of living beings, their fundamental essence combined in a very limited array of nucleic acids used as building blocks. In the race-blind, gender blind society of GATTACA, genetics suffices to validate a person's worth.

All of these essays make use of the privileged nature of the gaze—often held somehow to be a more objective means of depicting human conditions, less subject to the whims and fancies of the creator than mere words. Yet all three of these essays belie such a simplistic assumption. Behind the seeming transparency of visual images lies considerable opacity, as well as hidden choices by both artist and subject.

The choices made by Lam Qua are nicely explicated. Although these depictions were created before the widespread use of the photograph, we cannot help but view these images through the eyes of readers accustomed to photographs, movies, and video; it is easy to forget how carefully the artist must have had to plan each staging. The illusion of choice is perhaps greater here than in the photographs examined by Goler. Painting gave Lam Qua more flexibility, more ability to capture an exact moment than was possible with the slow film and lenses used to make the photographs of the day.

But it is not only the artist who wields power over how the image is to look; the patient, too, has some hidden power. Some of Lam Qua's subjects withhold their gaze, simply refusing to acquiesce to the desire to turn them into medical images. Although perhaps rare in the usual, canonical set of medical images, such behavior reappeared at the end of the nineteenth century when a new means of creating images came into being, an invention designed to see within the body. After the invention of the X-ray machine in 1895, many women feared the overly intrusive rays. State legislatures are said to have introduced legislation to ban the use of X-rays in public places, and enterprising entrepreneurs even offered lead-lined underwear for sale.

The power to hide is less obvious in the photographs of the American War between the States, where the gaze encompasses the new technologies of writing and counting, and—perhaps more importantly— is linked to the new technology and ideas about pensions and the role of state to provide for the wounded. The essence of GATTACA is the inability to hide. It is a world of invisible wounds, of inner genetic problems (located in this instance in a white male) being made manifest by the very lack of perfection, of standardization. The whole idea is to "pass" as something one is not, to modify one's physical appearance so as to "hide" the genetic truth, but even radical procedures to alter the outward appearance will not suffice. The medium for GATTACA, film, is both somehow more "realistic" and also an easier visual medium to reproduce (for showing in theaters or on home equipment) than Lam Qua's paintings. The medical museum, with its cases and boxes and labels and numbers, bridges the oil-painted world of Lam Qua to the organized genomic world of the twenty-first century.

CONTRIBUTORS

Lisa Diedrich is an assistant professor of women's studies at Stony Brook University. She is currently working on a book entitled *Treatments: Negotiating Bodies, Language, and Death in Illness Narratives.*

Sander L. Gilman is Distinguished Professor in the College of Liberal Arts and Sciences and the College of Medicine at the University of Illinois in Chicago. He is the director of the Humanities Laboratory and the first director of the Jewish Studies Program there. A cultural and literary historian, he is the author or editor of over seventy books. His first biography, *Jurek Becker: A Life in Five Worlds*, appeared in 2003 and his monograph *Fat Boys: A Slim Book* appeared in 2004; his most recent edited volume, *A Jew in the New Germany—Selected Writings of Henryk Broder* (with Lilian Friedberg), appeared that same year. He is the author of the basic study of the visual stereotyping of the mentally ill, *Seeing the Insane*, published by John Wiley and Sons in 1982 (reprinted in 1996) as well as the standard study of *Jewish Self-Hatred*, the title of his Johns Hopkins University Press monograph of 1986.

Robert I. Goler, an assistant professor of arts management at American University in Washington DC, has published widely on medical history. He is a recipient of the Lawrence D. Redway Award for Excellence in Medical History Writing from the Medical Society of the State of New York.

Joel Howell is the Victor Vaughan Professor of the History of Medicine at the University of Michigan, where he is also a practicing physician as well as the director of the Clinical Scholars Program. His research focuses on the role of medical technology in clinical medicine.

David A. Kirby has a PhD in evolutionary genetics and postdoctoral training in science and technology studies with scientific publications in the *Proceedings of the National Academy of Sciences* and *Genetics*. *Social Studies of Science*, *Public Understanding of Science*, and *Science Fiction Studies* have published his research on science communication and fiction. He is currently Lecturer in Science Communication at the Centre for the History of Science, Technology, and Medicine at the University of Manchester.

Thomas W. Laqueur teaches history at the University of California, Berkeley. His books include *Making Sex: Body and Gender from the Greeks to Freud* and *Solitary Sex: A Cultural History of Masturbation.*

Jonathan M. Metzl is an assistant professor of psychiatry and women's studies and director of the Culture, Health, and Medicine Program at the University of Michigan. In this capacity he works as an attending physician in the adult psychiatric clinics and teaches courses at the undergraduate and graduate levels. He has written for the *American Journal of Psychiatry*, the *Harvard Review of Psychiatry, Academic Medicine, Gender and History, Social Science and Medicine, Ms. Magazine,* and *SIGNS: The Journal of Women, Culture, and Society.* His book, *Prozac on the Couch: Prescribing Gender in the Era of Wonder Drugs,* was published in 2003 by Duke University Press.

Suzanne Poirier is a professor of literature and medical education and the director of Medical Humanities at the University of Illinois at Chicago College of Medicine. She is a past editor of *Literature and Medicine,* and she has published extensively in the areas of narrative and literature in medicine. Her work includes *Writing AIDS: Literature, Language, and Analysis* (coedited with Timothy F. Murphy); *Chicago's War against Syphilis: The Times, the* Trib, *and the Clap Doctor;* and *Stories of Family Caregiving: Reconsiderations of Theory, Literature, and Life* (coauthored with Lioness Ayres). She is currently working on a book-length study of memoirs of medical education.

Stephen Rachman teaches English at Michigan State University where he has directed the American Studies Program. He is currently the 2003–04 William S. Vaughn Visiting Fellow at the Robert Penn Warren Center for the Humanities at Vanderbilt University where he is working on a book on Peter Parker and Lam Qua. Most recently, he is a coauthor of *Cholera, Chloroform, and the Science of Medicine: A Life of John Snow* (Oxford 2003).

Tobin Siebers is V. L. Parrington Collegiate Professor of Literary and Cultural Criticism and the director of the Program in Comparative Literature and of the Global Ethnic Literatures Seminar. He is completing a book on disability studies called *Disability Theory.*

Sidonie Smith is the Martha Guernsey Colby Collegiate Professor of English and Women's Studies and chair of the Department of English at the University of Michigan. She was recently director of Women's Studies at Michigan. Her fields of interest include feminist theories, women's studies in literature, and autobiography studies. She is the author of *Human Rights and Narrated Lives: The Ethics of Recognition* (with Kay Schaffer, forthcoming, Palgrave, 2004); *Reading Autobiography: A Guide to Interpreting Personal Narratives* (with Julia Watson, 2001)); *Moving Lives: Women's Twentieth Century Travel Narratives,* (2001); *Subjectivity, Identity, and the Body: Women's Autobiographical Practices in the Twentieth Century* (1993); *A Poetics of Women's Autobiography: Marginality and the Fictions of Self-Representation* (1987); and *Where I'm Bound: Patterns of Slavery and Freedom in Black American Autobiography* (1974). She has coedited seven books, most recently *Inter/Faces: Women, Autobiography, Image, Performance* (with Julia Watson, 2002); and *Women, Autobiography, Theory: A Reader* (with Julia Watson, 1998). She has received fellowships at Canterbury Christ Church University College in New Zealand; the Humanities Research Centre at the Australian National University; and the Curtin University of Technology in Perth. Most recently, she was the Northrop Frye Fellow in Comparative Literatures at the University of Toronto.

Susan Squier received her education at Princeton University and Stanford University. She is now Brill Professor of Women's Studies and English at the Pennsylvania State University. Research interests include cultural studies of science and medicine, disability studies, feminist theory, and modernism. Major publications include *Virginia Woolf and London: The Sexual Politics of the City* (1985); *Babies in Bottles: Twentieth Century Visions of Reproductive Technology* (1994); *Women Writers and the City: Essays in Feminist Literary Criticism* (1984); *Arms and the Woman: War, Gender, and Literary Representation* (1989); *Playing Dolly: Technocultural Formations, Fantasies, and Fictions of Assisted Reproduction* (1999); *Communities of the Air: Radio Century, Radio Culture* (Duke University Press 2003); and *Liminal Lives: Imagining the Human at the Frontiers of Biomedicine* (forthcoming, Duke University Press, 2004). She was scholar in residence at the Rockefeller Foundation Bellagio Study and Conference Center (February–March 2001); Visiting Distinguished Fellow, LaTrobe University, Melbourne Australia (1992); and Fulbright Senior Research Scholar, Melbourne, Australia (1990–1991). She is on the editorial board of the *Journal of Medical Humanities* and executive board member and past president of the Society for Literature and Science. In the summer of 2002, she codirected (with Anne Hunsaker Hawkins) the NEH Summer Institute, "Medicine, Literature, and Culture," held at the Penn State College of Medicine, Hershey Medical Center.

Gregory Tomso received his PhD from Duke University in 2001 and is an assistant professor of English at Ithaca College. He is currently working on a book called *A Great Adventure: Leprosy, Stigma, and the Making of U.S. Culture*.

Sue Sun Yom is a resident in training in radiation oncology. She received an MD-PhD from the University of Pennsylvania in 2002. Her doctoral work was in English literature. Her interests include Virginia Woolf, Asian American fiction and film, cultural studies, and the medical humanities.